Oral Diagnosis

Petra Wilder-Smith • Janet Ajdaharian
Editors

Oral Diagnosis

Minimally Invasive Imaging Approaches

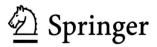 Springer

Editors
Petra Wilder-Smith
Beckman Laser Institute
University of California
Irvine School of Medicine
Irvine
CA
USA

Janet Ajdaharian
Chao Family Comprehensive Cancer
Center, University of California
Irvine School of Medicine
Irvine
CA
USA

ISBN 978-3-030-19252-5   ISBN 978-3-030-19250-1   (eBook)
https://doi.org/10.1007/978-3-030-19250-1

This Springer imprint is published by the registered company Springer Nature Switzerland AG
The registered company address is: Gewerbestrasse 11, 6330 Cham, Switzerland

Preface

The human race has made great progress in the quest to understand nature and harness its mysteries to improve our daily lives. It is fascinating, indeed, to note that our exploration at the extreme scales, from subatomic particles to distant galaxies, has a common vein: "light." Tremendous recent advances in optics and photonics are ushering in formidable new technologies, enabling personalized and precision medicine approaches to improve human health. This book represents an effort to provide a clinically focused overview of clinical applications of light in dentistry with an emphasis on clinical imaging techniques.

Optical imaging permits in vivo, real-time, non-perturbing, or minimally perturbing inspection of tissues, allowing safe and repeatable examination of biological tissues using non-ionizing imaging sources. Broadly speaking, optical imaging can be categorized as the ability of light to interrogate biological tissue by either diffusive (passive) or ballistic (active) interactions. The former modality is evident in interferometric approaches that largely depend on light reflection, refraction, and transmission, while the latter modalities are predominantly based on absorption, emission, excitation, as well as scattering. Some practical uses of these modalities include traditional intraoral cameras (digital dentistry), surgical loupes and microscopes, as well as laser Doppler techniques. Intraoral applications of new modalities such as optical coherence tomography (routinely used in ophthalmology), Raman spectroscopy, fluorescence imaging, photoacoustic imaging, and near-infrared spectroscopy have been investigated more recently. Ongoing advances in laboratory-based innovations such as super-resolution microscopy and multiphoton imaging still require translational efforts before they become suitable to human applications.

Among medical specialties, dentistry presents a challenging biological scenario where both hard (mineralized) and soft tissues play integral roles in enabling optimal craniofacial functions. The oral cavity is perhaps the best exemplar of all human mineralized hard tissues, with structural components ranging from the hardest known tissue, enamel, to the considerably softer dentin, cementum, bone, and cartilage. The oral soft tissues include specialized parakeratinized mucosa that provides resistance to physical (masticatory) compressive and shear forces, as well as non-keratinized lining mucosa. The latter includes specialized secretory glandular epithelium that produces saliva. There also exists an intermediate transitional epithelium between the oral mucosa and skin termed the vermillion (lip) border. A rather unique feature in the oral cavity, not present in any other anatomical site, is the anchoring of the tooth within a bony socket (alveolar bone) by means of a complex soft tissue (gingiva) and tooth attachment. This gingival attachment presents a unique mechanical, biological, and immunological niche that predominantly defines the progression of gingival and periodontal disease. Hence, these complex anatomical oral and dental structures present unique diagnostic challenges that require sophisticated hard and soft tissue imaging approaches to inform on and enable accurate interpretation of their health status, form, and structure.

The pathophysiological functions of the oral cavity involve an intricate interplay of the mechano-physical (occlusive, masticatory), fluid (saliva), immunological, and polymicrobial environment of the oral cavity. The latter, termed the oral *microbiome*, has opened new vistas in our understanding of oral-systemic health connections, giving new credence to the phrase the *oral health is a window into one's general health*. Imaging technologies that inform on the precise composition and functions of oral biofilm serve as powerful tools to gaining insights into its structure and function in healthy and pathological scenarios such as developmental anomalies, infections, injury, and malignancies. All of these necessitate early and precise diagnoses and monitoring.

An exciting future expansion of applications for innovative imaging modalities is the potential combinatorial approach of merging *thera*py with diag*nostics* termed *theranostics*. Therapeutic applications of biophotonics devices will potentially transform conventional restorative and prosthetic dentistry techniques through innovations such as direct combinatorial image-guided interventions and an exciting new focus on regenerative clinical dental applications. The innovations in optical and photonic technologies highlighted in this book provide clear evidence that clinical dentistry is well poised to play a leading role in healthcare innovation. The editors and contributors to this book are well known for their original contributions to the field of dental optical imaging. Overall, this book represents their sterling effort to showcase the current state of the art in optical imaging as applied to oral health. This book should be a very useful resource for dental clinicians and dental researchers alike in enabling safe, efficacious, and optimal oral health in the modern clinic.

Buffalo, NY, USA   Praveen R. Arany

Contents

Optical Methods for Monitoring Demineralization and Caries

Daniel Fried

Abstract

In this chapter optical methods for monitoring demineralization and remineralization on tooth coronal and root surfaces are presented. Methods discussed include transillumination and reflectance imaging with visible and near-IR light, fluorescence based imaging methods and optical coherence tomography (OCT). OCT can be used to acquire tomographic images of the structure of lesions in vivo and can be used to provide depth resolved measurements of the severity of demineralization. OCT can be used to detect if occlusal and proximal lesions have penetrated through the enamel to the underlying dentin. In addition, OCT can be used to monitor changes in lesion severity and presence of a transparent highly remineralized surface zone that is formed when lesions become arrested.

During the past century, the nature of dental decay or dental caries in the USA has changed markedly due to the introduction of fluoride to the drinking water, the advent of fluoride dentifrices and rinses, and improved dental hygiene. In spite of these advances, dental decay continues to be the leading cause of tooth loss in the USA [1–3]. By 17 years of age, 80% of children have experienced at least one cavity [4]. In addition two thirds of adults aged 35–44 years have lost at least one permanent tooth to caries. Older adults suffer tooth loss due to the problem of root caries. The nature of the caries problem has changed dramatically with the majority of newly discovered caries lesions being highly localized to the occlusal pits and fissures of the posterior dentition and the proximal contact sites between teeth. These early carious lesions are often obscured or "hidden" in the complex and convoluted topography of the pits and fissures or are concealed by debris that frequently accumulates in those regions of the posterior teeth. In the caries process, demineralization occurs as organic acids generated by bacterial plaque diffuse through the porous enamel of the tooth dissolving the mineral. If the decay process is not arrested, the demineralization spreads through the enamel and reaches the dentin where it rapidly accelerates due to the markedly higher solubility and permeability of dentin. The lesion spreads throughout the underlying dentin to encompass a large area, resulting in loss of integrity of the tissue and cavitation. Caries lesions are usually not detected until after the lesions have progressed to the point at which surgical intervention and restoration are necessary, often resulting in the loss of healthy tissue structure and weakening of the tooth. Therefore, new diagnostic tools are needed for the detection and characterization of caries

D. Fried (✉)
Division of Biomaterials and Bioengineering, Department of Preventive and Restorative Dental Sciences, University of California, San Francisco, San Francisco, CA, USA
e-mail: Daniel.Fried@ucsf.edu

© Springer Nature Switzerland AG 2020
P. Wilder-Smith, J. Ajdaharian (eds.), *Oral Diagnosis*, https://doi.org/10.1007/978-3-030-19250-1_1

lesions in the early stages of development. Carious lesions also occur adjacent to the existing restorations, and new tools are needed to diagnose the severity of those lesions and determine if an existing restoration needs to be replaced.

Caries lesions are routinely detected in the USA by using visual/tactile (explorer) methods coupled with radiography. These diagnostic and treatment paradigms were developed long ago and were adequate for large, cavitated lesions; however, they do not have sufficient sensitivity or specificity for the diagnosis of the early noncavitating caries lesions prevalent today. Radiographic methods do not have the sensitivity for early lesions, particularly occlusal lesions, and by the time the lesions are radiolucent, they have often progressed well into the dentin at which point surgical intervention becomes necessary [5]. At that stage in the decay process, it is far too late for preventive and conservative intervention and a large portion of carious and healthy tissue will need to be removed, often compromising the mechanical integrity of the tooth. If left untreated, the decay will eventually infect the pulp, leading to loss of tooth vitality and possible extraction. The caries process is potentially preventable and curable. If carious lesions are detected early enough, it is likely that they can be arrested/reversed by nonsurgical means through fluoride therapy, antibacterial therapy, dietary changes, or low-intensity laser irradiation [4, 6].

Accurate determination of the degree of lesion activity and severity is of paramount importance for the effective employment of the treatment strategies mentioned above. Since optical diagnostic tools exploit changes in the light scattering of the lesion, they have great potential for the diagnosis of the current "state of the lesion", i.e., whether or not the caries lesion is active and expanding or whether the lesion has been arrested and is undergoing remineralization. Therefore, new technologies are needed to determine whether caries lesions have been partially remineralized and have become arrested. Such data are also invaluable for caries management by risk assessment in the patient and for determining the appropriate form of intervention.

Conventional Methods of Caries Detection and Diagnostics

The most difficult to detect and the most common early enamel lesions are occlusal (biting surfaces) pit and fissure and approximal (contact surfaces between teeth) lesions. Occlusal lesions constitute 80% of the new lesions found today [7]. In the conventional method of occlusal caries detection, the clinician probes areas in the dentition that appear suspicious upon an initial visual inspection with the dental explorer [8]. If the probed area is soft and provides some resistance upon retraction of the instrument, the site is deemed to be carious. Studies suggest that the use of the dental explorer to probe for caries may actually promote or accelerate lesion formation [5, 9]. Thus, the use of a blunt explorer or none at all has been recommended by leading cariologists [10–12]. Clinicians base their diagnosis of occlusal lesions and treatment planning on the pit, fissure color, and texture. This can be misleading because lesion color does not provide sufficient information about the state of the lesion, i.e., whether it is progressing or arrested. Moreover, pigmentation can be due to staining from diet and other environmental factors and not from infection by microorganisms [13]. In a review of conventional methods of caries diagnosis, ten Cate [5] indicated that visual and tactile diagnosis of occlusal caries typically has a very low sensitivity ~0.3, implying that only 20–48% of the caries present (usually into the dentin) are found [5, 10, 14]. The specificity typically exceeds 0.95. The poor sensitivity can be attributed to the "hidden" nature of the majority of occlusal lesions. The bulk of the lesion is not accessible and is most often not detected unless it is so extensive that it is resolvable radiographically. New technology is needed that can detect these hidden areas of decay.

The International Caries Detection and Assessment System (ICDAS) was introduced several years ago [15, 16]. It is basically a diagnostic scoring system that relies on visual assessment. This system has been enthusiastically received and encourages more conservative dentistry; however, one should exercise caution regarding claims of high performance for caries detection and take into consideration that the system suffers from the limitations of visual assessment [17].

New radiographic methods employing digital imaging technology have higher sensitivity and use markedly reduced dosages of ionizing radiation to acquire diagnostic images [18]. Digital subtraction radiography can be used to monitor changes in mineral content in vitro [19]. However, since we still do not understand the risk of low-level exposure to ionizing radiation, even greatly reduced levels of radiation exposure may pose a significant risk. The principal limitation of bitewing radiographs for early caries detection is that they cannot be used to detect early occlusal caries lesions because of the overlapping features of the crowns. It is unlikely that improvements in radiographic sensitivity will enable detection of early enamel lesions because of this problem.

FOTI, DIFOTI, Proximal, and Occlusal Transillumination

Optical transillumination was used extensively before the discovery of X-rays for the detection of dental caries. Bitewing radiographs are the standard method of detection for approximal lesions. Unfortunately, as much as 25% of the proximal areas of bitewing X-rays are unresolved due to the overlap with healthy tooth structure on adjoining teeth, and X-rays typically underestimate the true depth of approximal lesions [20, 21]. Visual and radiographic methods have poor sensitivity (0.38 and 0.59) for approximal lesions, particularly noncavitated lesions and typically underestimate lesion severity [22].

The development of high-intensity fiber-optic light sources a few decades ago revived interest in optical transillumination for the detection of approximal lesions [20, 23–26]. During fiber-optic transillumination (FOTI), a carious lesion appears dark upon transillumination because of decreased transmission due to increased scattering and absorption by the lesion. A digital fiber-optic transillumination system, DiFoti (electro-optics sciences) that utilizes visible light for the detection of caries lesions was developed several years ago [27]. However, this system operated in the visible range where light scattering in enamel is high and the performance was limited. Near-IR light can penetrate a factor of 30 times further through the tooth enamel without scattering for markedly better performance [28, 29]. Light scattering in dental enamel decreases

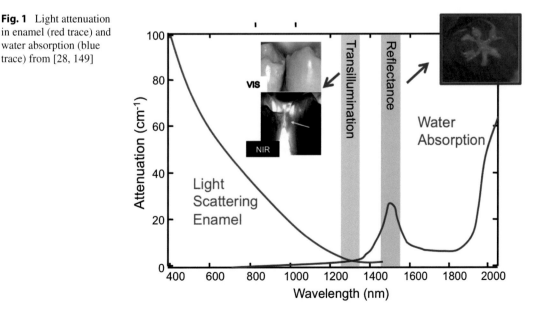

Fig. 1 Light attenuation in enamel (red trace) and water absorption (blue trace) from [28, 149]

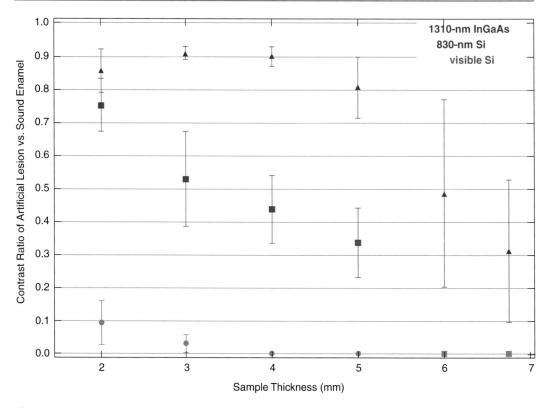

Fig. 2 Mean lesion contrast ($n = 3$) for simulated caries lesions in human enamel as a function of thickness for 1310, 830, and visible wavelengths from [34]

with increasing wavelength and enamel is the most transparent near $\lambda = 1300$ nm. A plot of the attenuation of light in enamel and water is shown in Fig. 1 as a function of wavelength from 400 to 2000 nm. The mean free path of light, i.e., how far it travels before being scattered or absorbed, is ~100 μm around $\lambda = 500$ nm and increases to between 3 and 4 mm near $\lambda = 1300$ nm [28, 29]. Moreover, optical property measurements of artificial and natural caries lesions show that the scattering of such lesions increases by 2–3 orders of magnitude upon demineralization at $\lambda = 1300$ nm, indicating that the highest contrast in transillumination between sound and carious tissues is found near $\lambda = 1300$ nm as well [30]. The contrast of simulated lesions in sections of enamel from 2 to 7 mm thickness is plotted in Fig. 2 for visible, 830 nm, and 1310 nm. The contrast is higher at 830 nm than the visible but the contrast is highest at 1310 nm, and only at

1310 nm is the lesion visible through 6–7 mm of enamel. Approximal [31] and occlusal lesions [32] can be imaged in whole teeth using near-IR 1310 nm light sources and an InGaAs imaging camera.

Due to the high transparency of enamel in the near-IR, novel imaging configurations are feasible in which the tooth can be imaged from the occlusal surface after shining light at and below the gumline, which we call occlusal transillumination [32, 33]. Approximal lesions can be imaged by occlusal transillumination of the proximal contact points between teeth and by directing near-IR light below the crown while imaging the occlusal surface [31, 33, 34]. The latter approach is capable of imaging occlusal lesions as well with high contrast [32, 33, 35–38].

Stains that are common on tooth occlusal surfaces do not interfere at longer near-IR wavelengths since none of the known chromophores absorb light at longer wavelengths. The photon energy is not sufficient for electronic excitation of the chromophores [32, 39]. Almaz et al. demonstrated that it is necessary to use near-IR wavelengths greater than 1150 nm to avoid significant interference from stains when measuring lesion contrast in reflectance and transillumination modalities [40]. Therefore stains can be easily differentiated from actual demineralization in the near-IR range, which is not possible at visible wavelengths. Chung et al. [41] demonstrated that absorption due to stains contributed more to the lesion contrast than increased scattering due to demineralization at visible wavelengths [42]. Since it is impractical to remove stains from the deep grooves and fissures on tooth occlusal surfaces, lack of interference from stains at longer near-IR wavelengths is a significant advantage.

In 2009, it was demonstrated that approximal lesions that appeared on radiographs could be detected in vivo with near-IR imaging with similar sensitivity [33] and that occlusal transillumination could be employed clinically. This was the first step in demonstrating the clinical potential of near-IR imaging for approximal caries detection. Figures 3 and 4 show radiographs and proximal and occlusal transillumination images of lesions acquired at 1310 nm from that study. Even though the sensitivity of radiographs is not very high [21, 22, 43–45], most studies indicate that the specificity of radiographs is above 90%, which makes it a suitable standard for comparison with the first test of this new imaging technology. In addition to demonstrating that the sensitivity of near-IR transillumination was as high as radiography, multiple imaging geometries were employed to aid in diagnosis, and it was shown that the occlusal transillumination imaging geometry in which light is applied near the gumline is extremely valuable for detecting approximal lesions [33]. In a second study com-

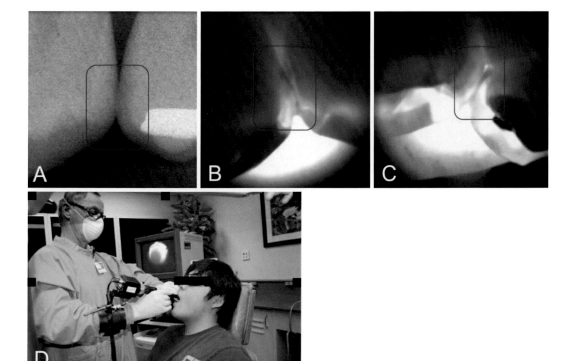

Fig. 3 Images from the first near-IR clinical imaging study. (**a**) radiograph, (**b**) near-IR proximal transillumination at 1310 nm (buccal view), (**c**) near-IR proximal transillumination at 1310 nm (lingual view), (**d**) picture of the imaging system in use [33]

Fig. 4 Near-IR occlusal transillumination images from the first near-IR clinical imaging study. Matching radiographs (left) and occlusal transillumination images at 1310 nm (right) are shown [33]

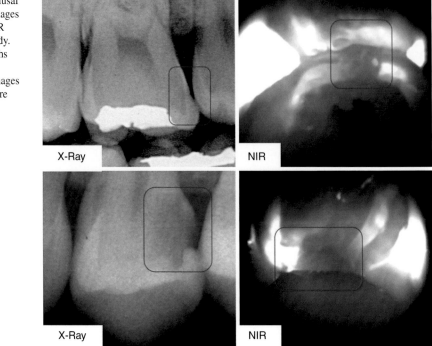

pleted in 2011, teeth with non-cavitated occlusal caries lesions that were not radiopositive were examined in test subjects using near-IR occlusal transillumination at 1300 nm prior to restoration [46]. That study demonstrated that occlusal caries lesions can be imaged with high contrast in vivo and that near-IR occlusal transillumination is an excellent screening tool for occlusal lesions.

In the most recent clinical study [47] at wavelengths greater than 1300 nm, the diagnostic performance of both near-IR transillumination and near-IR reflectance probes were used to screen premolar teeth scheduled for extraction. The teeth were collected and sectioned and examined with polarized light microscopy and transverse microradiography which served as the gold standard. In addition, extraoral radiographs of teeth were taken, and the diagnostic performance of near-IR imaging was compared with radiography. Near-IR imaging was shown to be significantly more sensitive than radiography for the detection of lesions on both occlusal and proximal tooth surfaces in vivo. The sensitivity of the combined near-IR imaging probes was signifi-

cantly higher ($P < 0.05$) than radiographs for both occlusal and proximal lesions in vivo. It was anticipated that near-IR methods would be more sensitive than radiographs since the radiographic sensitivity for occlusal lesions is extremely poor; however, the sensitivity was also much higher for approximal lesions than radiography, 0.53 vs. 0.23. In addition, the sensitivity of each individual near-IR method was either individually equal to or higher than radiography.

The first commercially available near-IR imaging device called the Diagnocam or CariesVu from Kavo (Biberach, Germany) uses an occlusal transillumination probe with 780 nm light [48, 49]. The shorter wavelength allows the use of less expensive silicon-based detectors. A previous in vitro study indicated that transillumination imaging at 830 nm with a low-cost silicon sensor optimized for the near-IR was capable of higher performance than visible systems, but the contrast was significantly lower than at 1300 nm and simulated lesions could not be imaged through the full enamel thickness [34]. It is also important to point out that stains are still highly visible at 780 nm [40].

Reflectance Imaging

Early enamel white spot lesions can be discriminated from sound enamel by visual observation or by visible-light diffuse reflectance imaging [50, 51]. Very early lesions can be detected visually. However, color, in addition to the intensity of the reflected light, plays a large role in detecting those changes. Moreover, such changes are difficult to quantify, and the color of sound tooth structure varies markedly. Specular reflectance is also a problem since enamel has a high refractive index. However, the visibility of scattering structures on highly reflective surfaces such as teeth can be enhanced by using crossed polarizers to remove the glare from the surface [52, 53]. The contrast between sound and demineralized enamel can be further enhanced by depolarization of the scattered light in the area of demineralized enamel [35, 54]. A more difficult problem to overcome is visible light absorption due to stains. In a recent study of natural lesions on the occlusal surfaces of extracted teeth, the image contrast was actually negative as opposed to being positive in visible reflectance measurements, indicating that absorption due to stains contributed more than increased scattering due to demineralization to the lesion contrast [41]. This renders the method useless in areas that are subject to heavy staining, namely the occlusal surfaces where most lesions are likely to develop. In fact, visible light reflectance was proposed three decades ago for use in monitoring early demineralization on tooth surfaces but has proven to be unsuccessful due to the problems indicated above [51].

In the early 1980s, ten Bosch et al. [51] introduced an optical monitor that used optical fibers for reflectance measurements on tooth surfaces. The reflectivity increased from the lesion area with increasing mineral loss [55]. Using the Kubelka–Munk equations, Ko et al. [56] showed that the optical scattering power correlated with mineral loss and yielded improved results over reflectance measurements. Blodgett [57] measured the optical bidirectional reflectance distribution functions (BRDF) and bidirectional scattering distribution functions (BSDF) from the surfaces of human incisors at 632, 1054, and 3390 nm. Analoui et al. [58] showed that multispectral La∗b∗ color coordinates measured using a diode-array spectrometer in the region 380–780 nm did not correlate well with the depth of artificial lesions.

The contrast between sound and demineralized enamel is greatest in the near-IR due to the minimal scattering of sound enamel, and this can be exploited for reflectance imaging of early demineralization [30]. Wu et al. [59] reported that the contrast between early demineralization was significantly higher at 1310 nm than in the visible range. Zakian acquired hyperspectral reflectance images of occlusal caries lesions and demonstrated that multi-wavelength images could be used to aid diagnosis [39]. The highest contrast is achieved at longer near-IR wavelengths coincident with higher water absorption [60]. Water in the underlying dentin and surrounding sound enamel absorbs the deeply penetrating light and reduces the reflectivity in sound areas. In turn, this results in higher contrast between sound and demineralized enamel. Figure 5 shows three

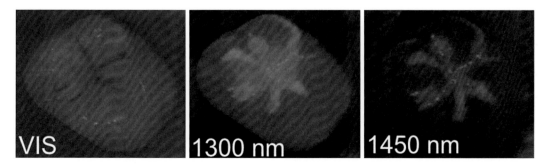

Fig. 5 Near-IR reflectance images of a tooth with stained fissures and demineralization at visible, 1300 nm, and 1450 nm

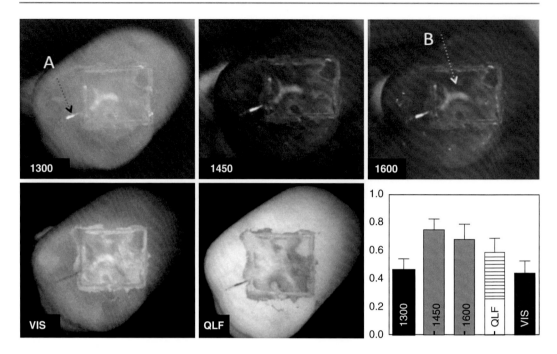

Fig. 6 Near-IR reflectance images at 1300, 1450, 1600 and in the visible and QLF of artificial lesions on the occlusal surface of a tooth. The mean (±SD) of the lesion contrast for 12 teeth is also shown, from [60]. The arrows labeled A and B point to an area of preexisting demineralization in the occlusal groove and the area of most severe demineralization that can be better differentiated in the near-IR images

reflectance images at visible wavelengths, 1300, and 1450 nm [41]. The highest contrast is at 1450 nm where there is a water absorption band. Note that the contrast is negative at visible wavelengths where absorption by stain dominates. Hyperspectral reflectance measurements by Zakian show that the tooth appears darker with increasing wavelength [39]. Figure 6 shows that the contrast of shallow demineralization in tooth occlusal surfaces is highest at 1450 nm and is significantly higher than QLF [60]. Recently a commercial near-IR reflectance system operating at 850 nm was introduced, Vistaproof from Durr Dental (Bietigheim-Bissingen, Germany). The first clinical study using near-IR reflectance was recently published, the wavelength range of 1500–1700 nm was used, and the diagnostic performance was higher than radiography and other near-IR imaging modalities for the detection of proximal and occlusal lesions [47].

Recent studies have shown that very high lesion contrast can be attained for very shallow lesions by using shorter wavelength blue light [61]. Blue light is scattered to a greater degree in

sound enamel than longer wavelengths in the visible and near-IR [28, 62, 63]. Monte Carlo simulations suggest that the optimal spectral region for the highest lesion contrast depends on the lesion depth and severity and that shorter wavelengths are likely to yield higher contrast for shallow lesions while longer wavelengths should yield higher contrast for deeper lesions [61].

An imaging method that shows a concomitant increase in lesion contrast with increasing lesion severity is more useful since the lesion severity can more easily be estimated from the images. Near-IR reflectance at wavelengths coincident with higher water absorption produced the greatest range of lesion contrast values and the contrast increased linearly with increasing lesion depth and severity [64].

Red or Porphyrin Fluorescence

Teeth naturally fluoresce upon irradiation with UV and visible light. Alfano [65] and Bjelkhagen et al. [66] demonstrated that laser-induced fluo-

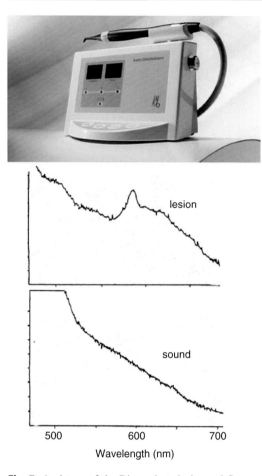

Fig. 7 A picture of the Diagnodent device and fluorescence spectra of sound and carious tooth structure adapted from Koenig et al. [150]

rescence (LIF) of endogenous fluorophores in human teeth could be used as a basis for discrimination between carious and noncarious tissues. Bacteria produce significant amounts of porphyrins and dental plaque fluoresces upon excitation with red light [67]. The earliest fluorescence measurements of dental caries showed the distinctive salmon red fluorescence due to porphyrins [65, 66]. Figure 7 shows fluorescence spectra of sound and carious areas of a tooth, with the characteristic salmon red porphyrin fluorescence from the lesion area. The first commercial system to exploit red fluorescence was the Diagnodent from Kavo (Biberach, Germany). The original device, shown in Fig. 7, uses a red diode laser and a fiber-optic probe designed to detect the fluorescence emitted from porphyrins at longer wavelengths. The probe is designed to

be inserted in an occlusal pit and fissure, and an electronic reading is generated representing the amount of fluorescence from the lesion. Bacteria produce significant amounts of porphyrins, and dental plaque fluoresces upon excitation with red light [67]. This device is designed to detect hidden occlusal lesions that have penetrated into the dentin where the high porosity concentrates porphyrins from bacteria. It is important to note that the primary microorganism responsible for dental decay, *Streptococcus mutans* does not contain porphyrins and that this method is not an effective means of monitoring cariogenic bacteria. Moreover, this device is designed to detect lesions in the later stage of development after the lesion has penetrated into the dentin and accumulated a considerable amount of bacterial byproducts. The Diagnodent has a poor sensitivity (~0.4) for lesions confined to enamel [68] since porphyrins have not accumulated in those lesions, and it is not capable of providing quantitative measurements of demineralization. An approximal caries probe designed to reach proximal surfaces has also been developed [69]. The Diagnodent is well-designed for the detection of "hidden" dentinal caries but does not provide quantitative measurements of demineralization [12].

Quantitative Light Fluorescence (QLF) (Green or Collagen Fluorescence)

QLF is the most extensively investigated optical technique for the measurement of surface demineralization. Ten Bosch [70] has described the mechanism for the QLF phenomenon, i.e., the loss of yellow/green fluorescence under illumination with blue light, and it can be solely explained by light scattering effects. Lesion areas appear dark due to increased light scattering in the lesion area that prevents the fluorescence from the underlying collagen in dentin or unknown fluorophores in enamel that are deeper in the tooth from reaching the tooth surface. Excitation wavelengths have varied from 370 to 488 nm, and blue laser diodes at 405 nm are more typically employed today. According to Kasha's rule,

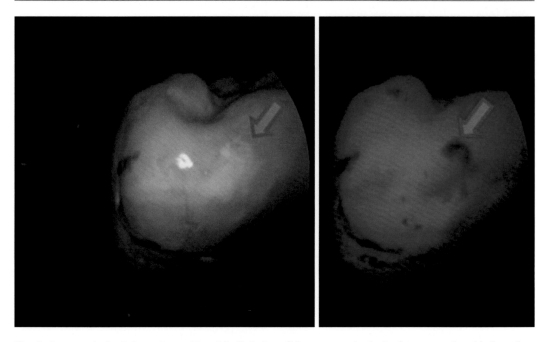

Fig. 8 Images obtained from the multimodal clinical device. (**a**) A 405 nm reflectance image with high resolution and contrast of the enamel surface. (**b**) The AF image of the same tooth obtained concurrently with the reflectance image. The arrows indicate a region with early caries from [151]

emission spectra are typically independent of excitation wavelength as long as the energy is high enough for excitation [71]. Fluorescence images provide increased contrast between sound and demineralized tooth structure and avoid the interference caused by specular reflection or high glare from the tooth surface that can interfere with visual detection of white spot lesions. An example of QLF images from a tooth with demineralization is shown in Fig. 8.

Hafstrom-Bjorkman et al. [72] established an experimental relationship between the loss of fluorescence intensity and the extent of enamel demineralization [72]. The method was subsequently labeled the QLF method, for quantitative laser fluorescence. An empirical relationship between overall mineral loss (ΔZ) vs. fluorescence loss was established which can be used to monitor lesion progression on enamel surfaces [73–75]. The gold standard for quantifying lesion severity and tooth surface and subsurface demineralization is transverse microradiography. The lesion severity is typically reported as the product of the volume % mineral loss and the lesion depth, ΔZ (vol.% × μm). Therefore, it is advantageous to be able to report a similar measure using optical methods. It is important to point out that QLF researchers report changes in fluorescence radiance ($\Delta F\%$) calculated as follows: $\Delta F_{Ref} = (F_{Ref}$ (demin)/F_{Ref} (sound)) × 100 for comparison with the ΔZ value measured with microradiography. Excellent correlation has been established between ΔF and ΔZ for shallow uniform artificial lesions [72, 76]. Amaechi et al. [77] compared the loss of reflectivity with lesion depth as measured with optical coherence tomography to the loss of fluorescence measured with QLF and achieved a very high correlation, suggesting both experiments measure the same thing, namely increased light attenuation due to an increase in light scattering in the lesion. Ando et al. [78, 79] established that the ΔF_{Ref} intensity for similar lesions depends on the actual enamel thickness. That result suggests a very serious limitation for clinical implementation since the enamel thickness varies markedly with position on each tooth and from tooth to tooth. Another complication is that stains and plaque fluoresce strongly, greatly confounding detection. Therefore, QLF has not been successfully validated for quantifying surface demineralization in the pits and fissures of the occlusal surfaces where most lesions are found and has shown relatively low specificity in clinical studies on smooth surfaces [76].

QLF has also been used to quantify and measure remineralization both in vitro and in vivo [80]. Studies have shown optical changes in the fluorescence intensity after exposure of in vivo white spot lesions around orthodontic brackets to a remineralization solution or removal of the plaque retention device [81, 82]. However, since QLF cannot produce an image of the internal structure of the lesion, it cannot be used to determine if actual mineral repair has taken place or that the lesion simply eroded away after removal of the bracket from abrasive action.

In summary, QLF performs well on carefully produced shallow uniform lesions on smooth surfaces free of stains. However, such performance cannot be expected on highly convoluted occlusal surfaces or the complex structures of natural lesions. Moreover, stains, plaque, and developmental defects interfere with QLF.

Several clinical devices are commercially available that measure either red or green fluorescence or both including QLF systems from Inspektor Research Systems (Amsterdam), Soprolife from Acteon Group (Norwick, England), Spectra and CamX from AirTechniques (Melville, NY), VistaCam from Durr Dental (Bietigheim-Bissingen, Germany), and IS Series Cameras from Carestream Dental (Rochester, NY).

Other fluorescence imaging techniques that have been employed for caries detection include time-resolved fluorescence [83], multiphoton fluorescence [84], dye-enhanced fluorescence [85], confocal fluorescence [75, 86], and modulated fluorescence or luminescence. Confocal fluorescence has considerable promise for studying very early incipient caries lesions.

Optical Coherence Tomography for Imaging Dental Caries

Optical coherence tomography (OCT) is a noninvasive technique for creating cross-sectional images of internal biological structure [87]. The intensity of the reflected/backscattered light is measured as a function of its axial position in the tissue. Low coherence interferometry is used to selectively remove or gate out the component of backscattered signal that has undergone multiple scattering events, resulting in very high axial resolution. The primary advantages of OCT for acquiring depth-resolved images of biological tissue include the capability for high resolution (~10 μm) coupled with good penetration depth (several mm) and utilization of fiber-optic probes for in vivo imaging. Ultrasound allows good imaging depth but has poor resolution (>100 μm) and cannot be easily used on teeth due to the high acoustic impedance. Confocal microscopic methods offer very high resolution, 100s of nm, but have limited penetration depths of less than 200 μm. They are also expensive and too bulky to be used in vivo.

The one-dimensional analog of OCT, optical coherence domain reflectometry (OCDR) was first developed as a high-resolution optical ranging technique for the characterization of optical components [88, 89]. Huang et al. [90] combined transverse scanning with a fiber-optic OCDR system to produce the first OCT cross-sectional images of biological microstructure, similar to ultrasound images, called "b-scans" as shown in Fig. 9. The first images of the soft and hard tissue structures of the oral cavity were acquired by Colston et al. [91, 92]. Feldchtein et al. [93] presented high-resolution dual wavelength 830 and 1280 nm images of dental hard tissues, enamel and dentin caries, and restorations in vivo. OCT has also been combined with QLF [94].

OCT can be used to measure the reflectivity within dental hard tissues to a depth of up to 3–4 mm in enamel and 1–2 mm in dentin. Figure 9 shows a 3D OCT tomographic image of a 6 × 6 mm² area of a tooth occlusal surface with lesions in the fissures. The b-scan image shows position and depth, and the magnitude of the reflectivity or back-scattered light at each pixel is displayed in a gray scale false color image with white indicating high reflectivity and black low reflectivity. Two a-scans of reflectivity vs. depth are shown in sound and lesion areas. The reflectivity from the lesion is orders of magnitude higher than the sound reflectivity.

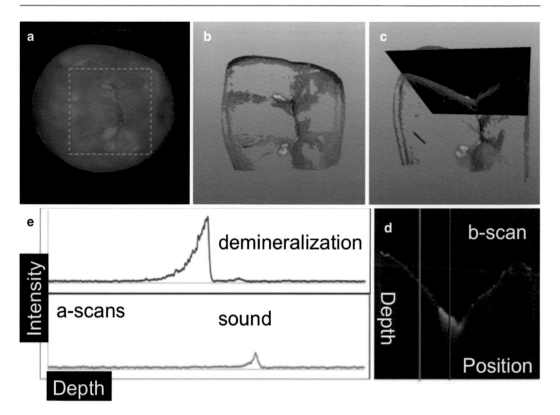

Fig. 9 A visible image of an extracted tooth (**a**) with demineralization in the fissure, a 5 × 5 mm box was cut to mark the ROI. (**b**, **c**) show the acquired CP-OCT 3D scans segmented to show areas of demineralization (red/yellow). A 2D slice extracted from the image at the position indicated in (**c**) is shown in (**d**), this is called a b-scan. The b-scan is displayed in grayscale with higher reflectivity in white which corresponds to demineralization. Two lineouts of depth vs intensity, called a-scans, were extracted (red and blue lines) at sound and lesion (demineralization) areas and are shown in (**e**)

High-speed Fourier domain systems (FD-OCT) are now available that can be operated with or without polarization sensitivity. For the older time-domain OCT systems (TD-OCT), the sensitivity (signal to noise) decreases markedly with increased scan rate, limiting the maximum scanning rate to 1–2 kHz. This is not a problem with the FD-OCT systems, where very high scanning rates can be achieved exceeding 100 kHz. Galvanometers or Microelectromechanical (MEMS) scanning mirrors can be used to scan the beam in two dimensions to acquire 3D images. This is a major step forward since entire 3D tomographic images can be acquired clinically, i.e., systems are capable of scanning at real-time video rates and are capable of acquiring images of a large area of the tooth without motion artifacts. However, at low scan rates, the performance of TD-OCT and FD-OCT systems are similar. In fact there are advantages to using TD-OCT for in vitro studies. In FD-OCT, a mirror image is generated by the Fourier transform so that more than half of the acquired image does not contain usable information. Therefore the number of data points acquired in each a-scan is lower for FD-OCT. Almost all the OCT systems available today utilize either swept-source (SS-OCT) or spectral domain (SD-OCT) systems. These systems were first used for dental imaging more than a decade ago [95–98]. SD-OCT systems are very popular for ophthalmology and for dermatology, but they have had limited applicability to dentistry since it is difficult to achieve axial resolutions exceeding 10 μm over scanning ranges greater than 2–3 mm. For dentistry, scanning ranges of 7 mm are needed to scan tooth occlusal surfaces and the high refractive index of enamel (1.63) further restricts the scanning range.

Methods for Assessing Lesion Severity with OCT and PS-OCT

Since OCT provides measurements of the optical reflectivity with depth, the most obvious method for quantifying the severity of demineralization in OCT images is to integrate the reflectivity over the lesion depth. However, the strong reflection at the tooth surface is typically several orders of magnitude higher than the reflectivity/scattering from the lesion itself, particularly for enamel. Moreover, this reflection from the surface varies markedly with angle of incidence, and the reflection can vary by several orders of magnitude. Therefore, it is problematic to use this value as a measure of lesion severity with a conventional OCT system. Because of this problem, the first attempts to use OCT to monitor demineralization utilized the loss of optical penetration as a measure of lesion severity. The loss correlated well with the mineral loss measured with microradiography for uniform artificial lesions on smooth surfaces [99]. Even though the loss of optical penetration can be invaluable for detecting shallow lesions in OCT images, there are major problems with using the loss of light penetration as a measure of lesion severity. One must arbitrarily choose a distance from the surface to serve as a cutoff point, based on an arbitrary intensity loss. This is feasible for smooth surfaces with uniform shallow lesions, but is not possible for highly convoluted surfaces, irregular lesion geometry or for lesions with significant structural variation. Moreover, OCT provides measurements of the reflectivity from each layer in the tissue. Since the reflectivity/scattering increases by 2–3 orders of magnitude in lesion areas due to an increase in light scattering, it is equally likely that there will be an increase in apparent optical penetration rather than a loss in signal especially for deep natural lesions or lesions in dentin, and one cannot assume that the underlying enamel is sound. More recently, other researchers with conventional OCT systems have used attenuation coefficients to quantify lesion severity [100, 101]. Both approaches are problematic since increased demineralization can lead to either an increase in attenuation of the reflectivity with depth or an increase due to the complex optical behavior. In

fact, this has led some researchers to mistakenly interpret the increase in apparent optical penetration of smooth surface lesions to indicate that the lesion is actually more transparent than the sound enamel [100]. In OCT images, it is easy to see deep strongly scattering tissues (lesions or dentin) below the weakly scattering sound enamel but not weakly scattering tissues under strongly scattering tissues.

Baumgartner et al. [102, 103] presented the first polarization resolved images of dental caries. PS-OCT images are typically processed in the form of phase and intensity images [53, 104], such images best show variations in the birefringence of the tissues. These early measurements indicated that it is advantageous to have polarization sensitivity to enhance the contrast of caries lesions and observe changes in birefringence that occur with demineralization. Later PS-OCT measurements demonstrated the advantage of using the cross-polarization OCT (CP-OCT) image to quantify lesion severity and track changes in lesion severity overtime [54]. Ko et al. showed that polarized Raman spectroscopy can be combined with OCT to help identify lesions [105, 106]. However, the polarization-dependent light scattering/reflectivity of PS-OCT provides the same information as polarization-dependent Raman scattering without requiring an additional Raman spectroscopy system. If the incident light is linearly polarized, surface reflections do not scramble the polarization, so the surface reflection does not interfere with the signal in the orthogonal ($\perp$) polarization state or CP image. Demineralization strongly scatters light increasing the light in the orthogonal polarization to the incident light [54]. Therefore, the reflectivity from lesion areas in the CP image can be directly integrated—including the very important surface zones near the tooth surface—thus overcoming the interference of strong surface reflections at tooth surfaces, a serious limitation of conventional OCT systems. Figure 10 shows PS-OCT b-scans across a fissure with a small lesion demonstrating the higher contrast of demineralization in the CP-OCT image. Enamel and dentin are birefringent tissues, so there is some reflectivity in the CP-image from sound tissues.

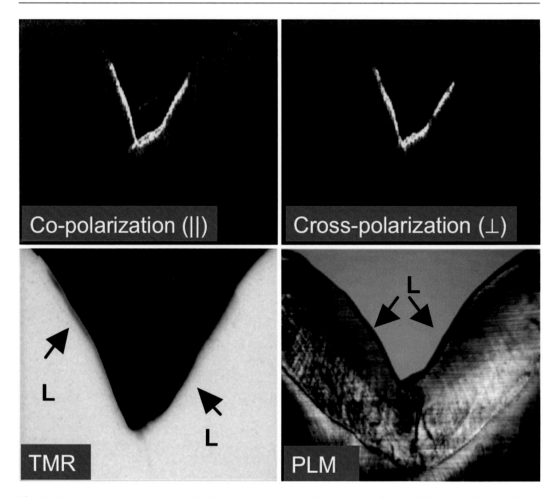

Fig. 10 Co-polarization and cross-polarization b-scans of demineralization in the fissure of the occlusal surface. Color table black < red < yellow < white < blue. PLM and TMR images are also shown for comparison, from [109]

The advantages of using PS-OCT to monitor demineralization and remineralization have been demonstrated in several studies utilizing various lesion models and natural lesions [36, 42, 54, 107–111]. The ability of PS-OCT to monitor remineralization and the formation of a distinct transparent surface zone [108, 112, 113] has also been demonstrated. Figure 11 shows PS-OCT co-polarization ($\parallel$) and cross-polarization ($\perp$) images of a bovine enamel sample with six windows showing sound, lesion, and lesion areas that have been exposed for 4, 8, and 12 days to a remineralization solution. There is minimal reflectivity in the sound regions outside the four windows, while the lesions have much higher contrast in the ($\perp$) or CP-OCT image. Although there was a high degree of remineralization, there was still

incomplete remineralization of the body of the lesion. The most obvious change was the formation of a distinct transparent outer surface layer 50 μm thick. The depth of the lesion shown in Fig. 11 was ~140 μm, and the depth did not decrease after remineralization. The integrated reflectivity for this sample decreased by ~50% after 12 days, showing less reflectivity from the body of the lesion [111].

PLM, $\perp$-axis PS-OCT, and TMR images of an occlusal lesion are shown in Fig. 12. Line profiles through different parts of the lesion were integrated to a depth of 500 μm for matching positions in the PS-OCT and TMR images to yield the integrated reflectivity, ΔR (dB × μm) and the integrated mineral loss ΔZ (vol.% × μm) for comparison. ΔR is analogous to ΔZ, the standard

Fig. 11 PS-OCT b-scan images of a bovine enamel block showing the sound (protected) regions located on the extreme left and right side of the sample, the lesion area (0 days exposed to remin. soln), and the areas exposed for increasing periods of time to the remineralization solution, 4, 8, and 12 days. The (‖) image represents the light reflected in the original polarization while the (⊥) image is the orthogonal polarization or cross-polarization image which was used for analysis in these studies. The incisions are ~100 μm deep and separated by 1.4 mm from [112]

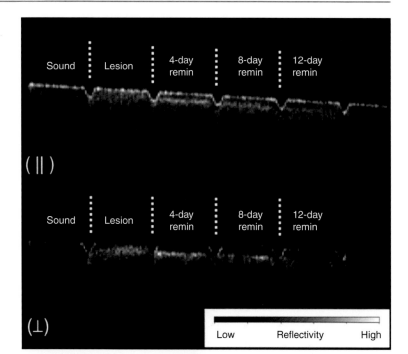

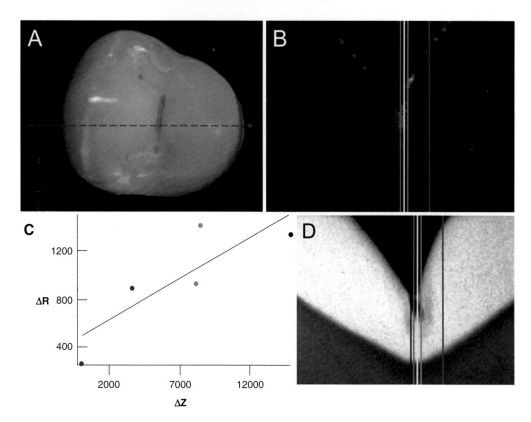

Fig. 12 A visible image of an extracted tooth (**a**), along with a CP-OCT b-scan taken at the position of the dashed arrow (**b**). In (**c**) the integrated reflectivity with depth (ΔR) from the CP-OCT scan and the integrated mineral loss over the lesion depth (ΔZ) from a matching trans-verse microradiograph taken of a thin section at the position of the dashed line in (**a**) which is shown in (**d**). Each colored data point in (**c**) was taken at the positions marked by the colored lines in (**b**) and (**d**)

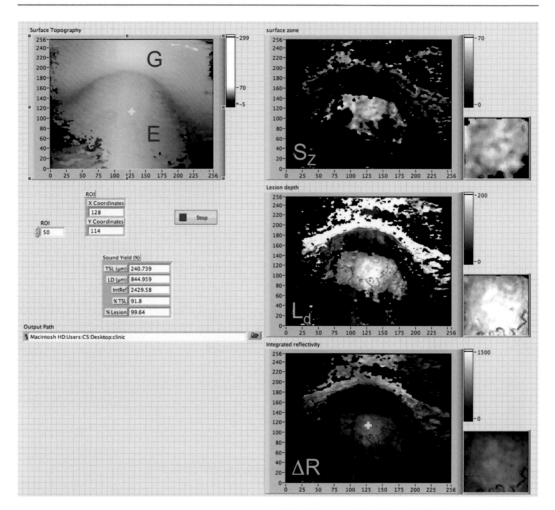

Fig. 13 Image of the front end of a program that our group developed for automated analysis of CP-OCT 3D images. Clinical data is shown for one lesion at a single time point. The image on the upper left shows a 2D image of the surface topography with intensity varying with height, the gingiva (G), and enamel (E) which is shown with the gingival margin in between. A lesion is located in the area of the yellow rectangular box in the S_z image. The three images on the right are the 2D images for the surface zone thickness (S_z), lesion depth (L_d), and integrated reflectivity over the lesion depth (ΔR), and the small boxes to the right of each image are those values for a specific ROI, in this case the 1 mm × 1 mm ROI was centered on the small yellow cross. Mean values are calculated for each ROI

unit used to represent lesion severity that is assessed using TMR [110, 114–117]. Five PS-OCT line profiles were taken at different positions in the lesion and integrated to yield ΔR and ΔZ, and there is excellent correlation.

Automated methods have been developed for converting 3D CP-OCT images to 2D projection images of the lesion depth (L_d), ΔR, and the thickness of the transparent surface zone (S_z) [110, 111]. Figure 13 shows processed in vivo images

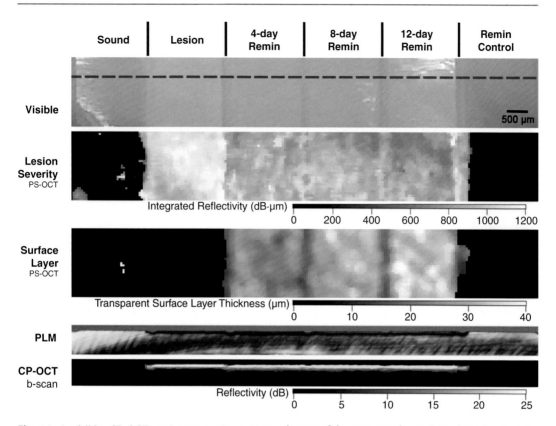

Fig. 14 A visible, CP-OCT, and cross-sectional PLM images of a bovine enamel sample with six windows. Initial lesions were produced after 24 h demineralization on the central four windows and then the right four windows were exposed to a remineralization solution. The red dotted line in the visible light reflectance image represents the position of the section shown in the PLM and CP-OCT images. Two-dimensional CP-OCT surface projection images of the same sample are shown including the integrated reflectivity (lesion severity) and the transparent surface layer thickness. PLM and processed CP-OCT b-scan images show an increase in transparent surface layer thickness over the periods of exposure to the remineralizing solution. The transparent surface layer is highlighted in yellow in the CP-OCT b-scan, from [111]

taken from a tooth with a cervical lesion created with a program for automated processing of the $6 \times 6 \times 7$ mm volumetric CP-OCT data. Images of the surface topography, as well as L_d, ΔR, and S_z are shown. A region of interest (ROI) was chosen for analysis, in this case a 1×1 mm box in the center of the lesion area shown in the small satellite boxes to the right of each image. The mean values of L_d, ΔR, and S_z in the box can be monitored over time to quantify changes in the lesion severity. Figure 14 shows a bovine enamel slab

$(10 \text{ mm} \times 2 \text{ mm} \times 2 \text{ mm})$ with six windows; the left and right windows are sound and in between are four windows for which the lesion has been exposed to remineralization for 0, 4, 8, and 12 days [111]. The 3D CP-OCT image was converted to 2D projection images of the integrated reflectivity over the lesion depth, ΔR, and the surface zone thickness, S_z. The decrease in the lesion severity with time is more accurate, and the growth of the surface zone can be clearly seen after exposure to a remineralization regimen.

Assessment of the Depth of Occlusal Lesions

Many clinicians are primarily interested in knowing how deep the occlusal lesions have actually penetrated into the tooth, so that they can decide whether a restoration is necessary. Recent studies utilizing the NIH-funded Practice-Based Research Network (http://www.nationaldentalp-brn.org) [118–120] indicated that a third of all patients have a questionable occlusal caries lesion (QOC) which can be defined as an occlusal tooth surface with no cavitation and no radiographic radiolucencies, but caries is suspected due to roughness, surface opacities, or staining. After monitoring QOCs for 20 months, 90% did not require intervention. The identification of occlusal lesions penetrating to dentin is poor with an accuracy of ~50% [121, 122]. OCT is ideally suited for monitoring and improving the diagnosis of QOCs, and methods can be developed to enhance the visibility of hidden subsurface lesions. Even though the optical penetration of near-IR light can easily exceed 7 mm through sound enamel to image lesions on proximal surfaces with high contrast [34], the large increase in light scattering due to demineralization [30] typically limits optical penetration in highly scattering lesions (also in dentin and bone) to 1–2 mm, thus cutting off the OCT signal before it reaches the dentinal–enamel junction (DEJ). Typically lesions spread laterally under the enamel upon contacting the more soluble softer dentin. Therefore, OCT can be used to determine if occlusal lesions have penetrated to the underlying dentin [46, 123] by detecting the lateral spread across the DEJ. In a clinical study, 12 out of 14 of the lesions examined in vivo using OCT exhibited increased reflectivity below the DEJ, indicating that the lesions had spread to the dentin. Since none of the lesions were visible on a radiograph, this demonstrates a remarkable improvement over existing technology [46, 123].

The visibility of QOCs can be significantly increased by the use of optical clearing agents and image analysis methods [124]. Optical clearing agents have routinely been used in biological microscopy and have found recent application in clinical imaging including OCT [125, 126]. Higher refractive index agents also appear to increase the optical penetration depth of OCT [127]. The viscosity is also important because penetration of the agent into the lesion pores can decrease the lesion contrast. Even though such penetration may lower the contrast of the lesion near the tooth surface, it increases the optical penetration to deeper layers in the lesion. In addition, various image analysis methods have been developed for enhancing the visibility of subsurface structures and edges, speckle reduction, and denoising OCT images [128–130]. The Rotating Kernel Transformation (RKT) is one approach that has been successful for edge detection in OCT images [111, 131–133]. In a recent study, extracted teeth with QOCs were imaged with optical coherence tomography (OCT) with and without the addition of a transparent vinyl polysiloxane impression material (VPS) that is commonly used in vivo. VPS acts as an optical clearing agent to enhance the visibility of occlusal lesions that have penetrated to the underlying dentin and also enhance the visibility of the dentinal–enamel junction (DEJ). Application of VPS significantly increased ($P < 0.0001$) the integrated reflectivity of subsurface dentinal lesions [124].

Assessment of Root Caries

Even though the penetration depth of near-IR light is more limited in dentin than for enamel, one can still acquire images of early root caries and demineralization in dentin [134]. PS-OCT studies have successfully measured demineralization in simulated caries models in dentin and on root surfaces (cementum) [135–137]. PS-OCT can effectively be used to discriminate demineralized dentin from sound dentin and cementum [135]. PS-OCT has also been used to measure remineralization on dentin surfaces and to detect the formation of a highly mineralized layer on the lesion surface after exposure to a remineralization solution [137]. Cementum has lower reflectivity than dentin in OCT images, making it possible to easily discriminate the remaining cementum thickness [135, 137]. Shrinkage occurs in demineralized dentin due to the high collagen content when the lesion area loses water. More severe lesions manifest greater shrinkage and lesions exposed to remineralization with an intact highly mineralized surface zone have reduced shrinkage [137]. There was a correlation between the lesion severity (ΔZ) and the degree of shrinkage measured using PS-OCT [138]. OCT has also been used to help discriminate between noncarious cervical lesions and root caries in vivo [139].

Assessment of Secondary Caries and Decay Under Sealants

OCT can be used to look at different restorative materials and identify pit and fissure sealants [93, 140]. The penetration depth of PS-OCT through composite has been shown to be sufficient to detect and track early demineralization or secondary caries on the occlusal surface under a sealant or restoration in vitro. The penetration depth is not greatly influenced by the composition of the filler. The reflectivity, however, is markedly increased when an optical pacifier such as titanium dioxide is added [107].

Most composites/sealants have sufficient transparency in the near-IR to allow imaging through the composite to resolve early demineralization under sealants and restorations. Polarization sensitivity may also help in identifying particular sealants since they apparently depolarize light at different rates. Jones et al. [107] showed that one particular sealant had minimal reflectivity in the orthogonal polarization image, i.e., does not depolarize the incident light and has minimal birefringence. The fact that there is minimal reflectivity from overlying composite also greatly facilitates direct integration of the reflectivity from the demineralized area. These images demonstrate that polarization sensitivity is advantageous for differentiating demineralized enamel under composite sealants and restorations for imaging secondary caries lesions. Other studies have investigated the use of OCT for the detection of demineralization beneath

sealants and composites in addition to primary lesions [141–145].

Clinical Studies Monitoring Demineralization/Remineralization

Feldchtein et al. [93] presented the first in vivo OCT images of dental caries. In the first clinical study using OCT to monitor demineralization, the development of demineralization on tooth occlusal and smooth surfaces was monitored [146]. Orthodontic bands with a buccal window were cemented on premolars, and small incisions were produced on occlusal surfaces to serve as sites for plaque retention for enhanced demineralization. Bands were removed after 30 days, and PS-OCT scans were acquired in vivo of occlusal and buccal areas, and ΔR was calculated from the CP-OCT images of the lesion areas. Teeth were extracted, serially sectioned, and analyzed using PLM and TMR for comparison with the CP-OCT images. PS-OCT was able to non-destructively measure significant increases in demineralization on both the buccal and occlusal surfaces [146]. In that study, a time-domain PS-OCT system was employed with a custom built handheld scanner shown in Fig. 15 that was capable of acquiring single b-scans in a few seconds over tooth buccal and occlusal surfaces. Difficulties in matching PS-OCT b-scans to the histological thin sections suggested that entire tomographic images (3D images) encompassing the entire lesion area should be acquired.

In a subsequent study, a high-speed swept-source CP-OCT system with an integrated MEMS scanner from Santec (Komaki Aichi, Japan) was used to acquire 3D volumetric images of the area at the base of orthodontic brackets over a period of 12 months after placement. The system and images from the study are shown in Fig. 16. The reflectivity was measured at 3-month intervals for 12 months to determine if there was increased demineralization. Even though an increase in demineralization was not visibly apparent in images taken before and after 12 months, CP-OCT was successful in monitoring a small but significant ($p < 0.05$) increase in

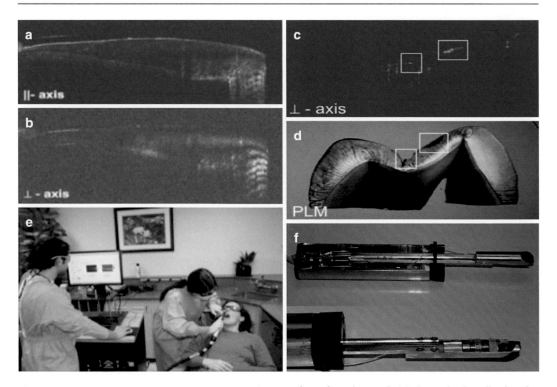

Fig. 15 Co-polarization (**a**) and cross-polarization (**b**). OCT b-scans of a sound area of the tooth from the first clinical study monitoring demineralization in vivo showing clear resolution of the dentinal–enamel junction from the crown to the root. The CP-OCT image of the occlusal surface of another tooth (**c**) shows demineralization that was confirmed using polarized light microscopy (**d**) after tooth extraction. The PS-OCT system is shown in use (**e**) along with images of the custom fabricated scanning probe (**f**) from [146]

the mean lesion depth (L_d) and integrated reflectivity (ΔR) with time over the area cervical to the brackets further validating the utility of CP-OCT for monitoring early demineralization [147].

In a clinical study recently completed, existing smooth surface enamel lesions were monitored using CP-OCT over a period of 30 weeks before and after application of a fluoride varnish [148]. Each lesion was imaged before application of the varnish and at 6-week intervals. It was interesting to observe that a transparent surface zone was visible in CP-OCT images for all but one of the enamel lesions (62/63). CP-OCT images from one test subject are shown in Fig. 17. A distinct surface zone approximately 150-μm thick is clearly visible. After 30 weeks, the lesion structure, depth, and severity (integrated reflectivity) remained the same, suggesting that this

lesion was already arrested. There was no significant change ($P > 0.05$) in L_d, ΔR, or the surface zone thickness (S_z) after 30 weeks for the 63 enamel lesions monitored. All 63 lesions were present after 30 weeks, and no changes were apparent upon clinical examination (photographs). Linear regression was used to determine if there was a significant increase in S_z with time for each lesion (positive slope significantly different from 0, $P < 0.05$), and only a small fraction of the lesions manifested a significant increase in S_z, 7 out of 63. Even though most of the lesions were likely arrested and underwent little change with intervention, the study demonstrated that the internal microstructure of caries lesions could be monitored overtime during preventative intervention. This ability offers many intriguing possibilities for future caries research.

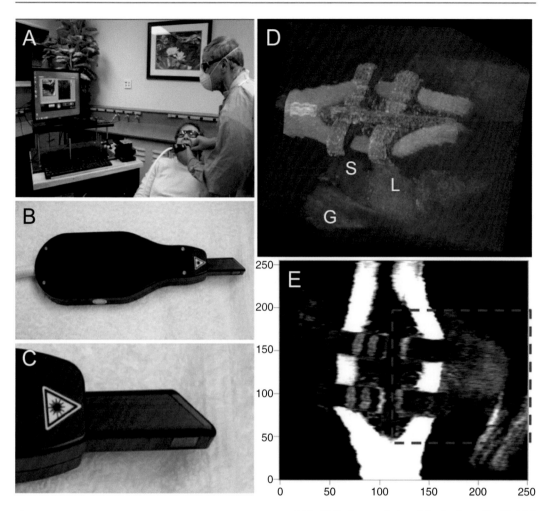

Fig. 16 Images from the first clinical study monitoring demineralization with a high-speed 3D CP-OCT system. The Santec system is shown in (**a**) along with the handpiece with integrated inteferometer and MEMS scanner in (**b**) and (**c**). (**d**) Surface rendering of 6 × 6 × 7 mm 3D CP-OCT image around bracket; G-gingiva, S-sound, and L-lesion. (**e**) Collapsed 2D image of ΔR (rotated by 90°) showing the area monitored over time in red box from [147]

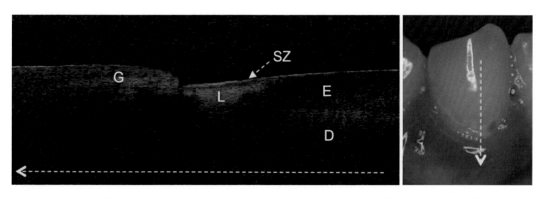

Fig. 17 An in vivo CP-OCT b-scan of a cervical enamel lesion that appears arrested. There was no change in the lesion structure after treatment with fluoride varnish after 30 weeks. The lesion is clearly visible, and it has a well-defined surface zone (S_Z) that is visible. The dentinal–enamel junction (DEJ) and the gingival (G) are visible in the image, and the position of the scans are indicated on the photograph of the tooth from [148]

References

1. Chauncey HH, Glass RL, Alman JE. Dental caries, principal cause of tooth extraction in a sample of US male adults. Caries Res. 1989;23:200–5.
2. Kaste LM, Selwitz RH, Oldakowski RJ, Brunelle JA, Winn DM, Brown LJ. Coronal caries in the primary and permanent dentition of children and adolescents 1-17 years of age: United States, 1988-1991. J Dent Res. 1996;75:631–41.
3. Winn DM, Brunelle JA, Selwitz RH, Kaste LM, Oldakowski RJ, Kingman A, Brown LJ. Coronal and root caries in the dentition of adults in the United States, 1988-1991. J Dent Res. 1996;75:642–51.
4. NIH. Diagnosis and management of dental caries throughout life: NIH consensus statement. Report nr 18; 2001. p. 1–24.
5. ten Cate JM, van Amerongen JP. Caries diagnosis: conventional methods. In: Early detection of dental caries. Bloomington: Indiana University; 1996. p. 27–37.
6. Featherstone JDB. Prevention and reversal of dental caries: role of low level fluoride. Community Dent Oral Epidemiol. 1999;27:31–40.
7. Dodds DJ. Dental caries diagnosis—toward the 21st century. Nat Med. 1996;2:281.
8. Carlos JP, Brunelle JA, editors. Oral health surveys of the NIDR: diagnostic criteria and procedures. NIH Publication No. 91-2870. Bethesda: U.S. Department of Health and Human Services; 1991.
9. Ekstrand K, Qvist V, Thylstrup A. Light microscope study of the effect of probing in occlusal surfaces. Caries Res. 1987;21(4):368–74.
10. Kidd EAM, Ricketts DNJ, Pitts NB. Occlusal caries diagnosis: a changing challenge for clinicians and epidemiologists. J Dent Res. 1993;21:3232–331.
11. Lussi A, Firestone A, Schoenberg V, Hotz P, Stich H. In vivo diagnosis of fissure caries using a new electrical resistance monitor. Caries Res. 1991;29:81–7.
12. Lussi A, Imwinkelreid S, Pitts NB, Longbottom C, Reich E. Performance and reproducibility of a laser fluorescence system for detection of occlusal caries in vitro. Caries Res. 1999;33:261–6.
13. Ekstrand K, Ricketts DNJ, Kidd EAM, Qvist V, Thylstrup A. Reproducibility and accuracy of three methods for assessment of demineralization depth on the occlusal surface. Caries Res. 1997;31:224–31.
14. Wenzel A. New caries diagnostic methods. J Dent Educ. 1993;57:428–32.
15. Ferreira Zandona A, Santiago E, Eckert G, Fontana M, Ando M, Zero DT. Use of ICDAS combined with quantitative light-induced fluorescence as a caries detection method. Caries Res. 2010;44(3):317–22.
16. Pitts N. "ICDAS"—an international system for caries detection and assessment being developed to facilitate caries epidemiology, research and appropriate clinical management. Community Dent Health. 2004;21(3):193–8.
17. Pitts N, editor. Detection, assessment, diagnosis and monitoring of caries, vol. 21. Basel: Karger; 2009.
18. Pitts N. Advances in radiographic detection methods and caries management rationale. In: Early detection of dental caries. Bloomington: Indiana University; 1996. p. 39–50.
19. Lenhard M, Mayer T, Pioch T, Eickholz P. A method to monitor dental demineralization in vitro. Caries Res. 1996;30:326–33.
20. Pine CM. Fiber-optic transillumination (FOTI) in caries diagnosis. In: Early detection of dental caries. Bloomington: Indiana University; 1996. p. 51–66.
21. Pine CM, ten Bosch JJ. Dynamics of and diagnostic methods for detecting small carious lesions. Caries Res. 1996;30(6):381–8.
22. Peers A, Hill FJ, Mitropoulos CM, Holloway PJ. Validity and reproducibility of clinical examination, fibre-optic transillumination, and bite-wing radiology for the diagnossis of small approximal carious lesions. Caries Res. 1993;27:307–11.
23. Peltola J, Wolf J. Fiber optics transillumination in caries diagnosis. Proc Finn Dent Soc. 1981;77:240–4.
24. Barenie J, Leske G, Ripa LW. The use of fiber optic transillumination for the detection of proximal caries. Oral Surg. 1973;36:891–7.
25. Holt RD, Azeevedo MR. Fiber optic transillumination and radiographs in diagnosis of approximal caries in primary teeth. Community Dent Health. 1989;6:239–47.
26. Mitropoulis CM. The use of fiber optic transillumination in the diagnosis of posterior approximal caries in clinical trials. Caries Res. 1985;19:379–84.
27. Schneiderman A, Elbaum M, Schultz T, Keem S, Greenebaum M, Driller J. Assessment of dental caries with digital imaging fiber-optic transillumination (DIFOTI): in vitro study. Caries Res. 1997;31:103–10.
28. Fried D, Glena RE, Featherstone JD, Seka W. Nature of light scattering in dental enamel and dentin at visible and near-infrared wavelengths. Appl Opt. 1995;34(7):1278–85.
29. Jones RS, Fried D. Attenuation of 1310-nm and 1550-nm laser light through sound dental enamel. In: Lasers in dentistry VIII. Proc SPIE vol. 4610; 2002. p. 187–190.
30. Darling CL, Huynh GD, Fried D. Light scattering properties of natural and artificially demineralized dental enamel at 1310-nm. J Biomed Optics. 2006;11(3):34023.
31. Jones RS, Huynh GD, Jones GC, Fried D. Near-IR transillumination at 1310-nm for the imaging of early dental caries. Opt Express. 2003;11(18):2259–65.
32. Buhler C, Ngaotheppitak P, Fried D. Imaging of occlusal dental caries (decay) with near-IR light at 1310-nm. Opt Express. 2005;13(2):573–82.
33. Staninec M, Lee C, Darling CL, Fried D. In vivo near-IR imaging of approximal dental decay at 1,310 nm. Lasers Surg Med. 2010;42(4):292–8.
34. Jones G, Jones RS, Fried D. Transillumination of interproximal caries lesions with 830-nm light.

In: Lasers in dentistry X. SPIE. vol. 5313; 2004. p. 17–22.

35. Fried D, Featherstone JDB, Darling CL, Jones RS, Ngaotheppitak P, Buehler CM. Early caries imaging and monitoring with near-IR light. Dent Clin North Am. 2005;49(4):771–94.

36. Hirasuna K, Fried D, Darling CL. Near-IR imaging of developmental defects in dental enamel. J Biomed Opt. 2008;13(4):044011.

37. Lee C, Lee D, Darling CL, Fried D. Nondestructive assessment of the severity of occlusal caries lesions with near-infrared imaging at 1310 nm. J Biomed Opt. 2010;15(4):047011.

38. Karlsson L, Maia AMA, Kyotoku BBC, Tranaeus S, Gomes ASL, Margulis W. Near-infrared transillumination of teeth: measurement of a system performance. J Biomed Opt. 2010;15(3):036001.

39. Zakian C, Pretty I, Ellwood R. Near-infrared hyperspectral imaging of teeth for dental caries detection. J Biomed Opt. 2009;14(6):-064047.

40. Almaz EC, Simon JC, Fried D, Darling CL. Influence of stains on lesion contrast in the pits and fissures of tooth occlusal surfaces from 800-1600-nm. In: Lasers in dentistry XXII. Proc SPIE. vol. 96920X; 2016. p. 1–6.

41. Chung S, Fried D, Staninec M, Darling CL. Multispectral near-IR reflectance and transillumination imaging of teeth. Biomed Opt Express. 2011;2(10):2804–14.

42. Chong SL, Darling CL, Fried D. Nondestructive measurement of the inhibition of demineralization on smooth surfaces using polarization-sensitive optical coherence tomography. Lasers Surg Med. 2007;39(5):422–7.

43. Purdell-Lewis DJ, Pot T. A comparison of radiographic and fibre-optic diagnoses of approximal caries lesions. J Dent. 1974;2(4):143–8.

44. Vaarkamp J, ten Bosch JJ, Verdonschot EH, Bronkhoorst EM. The real performance of bitewing radiography and fiber-optic transillumination in approximal caries diagnosis. J Dent Res. 2000;79(10):1747–51.

45. Stephen KW, Russell JI, Creanor SL, Burchell CK. Comparison of fibre optic transillumination with clinical and radiographic caries diagnosis. Community Dent Oral Epidemiol. 1987;15(2):90–4.

46. Staninec M, Douglas SM, Darling CL, Chan K, Kang H, Lee RC, Fried D. Nondestructive clinical assessment of occlusal caries lesions using near-IR imaging methods. Lasers Surg Med. 2011;43(10):951–9.

47. Simon JC, Lucas SA, Lee RC, Staninec M, Tom H, Chan KH, Darling CL, Fried D. Near-IR transillumination and reflectance imaging at 1300-nm and 1500-1700-nm for in vivo caries detection. Lasers Surg Med. 2016;48(6):828–36.

48. Kuhnisch J, Sochtig F, Pitchika V, Laubender R, Neuhaus KW, Lussi A, Hickel R. In vivo validation of near-infrared light transillumination for interproximal dentin caries detection. Clin Oral Investig. 2015;20(4):821–9.

49. Sochtig F, Hickel R, Kuhnisch J. Caries detection and diagnostics with near-infrared light transillumination: clinical experiences. Quintessence Int. 2014;45(6):531–8.

50. Angmar-Mansson B, ten Bosch JJ. Optical methods for the detection and quantification of caries. Adv Dent Res. 1987;1(1):14–20.

51. ten Bosch JJ, van der Mei HC, Borsboom PCF. Optical monitor of in vitro caries. Caries Res. 1984;18:540–7.

52. Benson PE, Ali Shah A, Robert Willmot D. Polarized versus nonpolarized digital images for the measurement of demineralization surrounding orthodontic brackets. Angle Orthod. 2008;78(2):288–93.

53. Everett MJ, Colston BW, Sathyam US, Silva LBD, Fried D, Featherstone JDB. Non-invasive diagnosis of early caries with polarization sensitive optical coherence tomography (PS-OCT). In: Lasers in dentistry V. SPIE. vol. 3593; 1999. p. 177–183.

54. Fried D, Xie J, Shafi S, Featherstone JDB, Breunig T, Lee CQ. Early detection of dental caries and lesion progression with polarization sensitive optical coherence tomography. J Biomed Optics. 2002;7(4):618–27.

55. Brinkman J, ten Bosch JJ, Borsboom PCF. Optical quantification of natural caries in smooth surfaces of extracted teeth. Caries Res. 1988;22:257–62.

56. Ko CC, Tantbirojn D, Wang T, Douglas WH. Optical scattering power for characterization of mineral loss. J Dent Res. 2000;79(8):1584–9.

57. Blodgett DW, Webb SC. Optical BRDF and BSDF measurements of human incisors from visible to mid-infrared wavelengths. Proc SPIE Int Soc Opt Eng. 2001;4257:448–54.

58. Analoui M, Ando M, Stookey GK. Comparison of Reflectance Spectra of Sound and Carious Enamel. In: Lasers in Dentsitry VI. SPIE. vol. 3910; 2000. p. 1017–2661.

59. Wu J, Fried D. High contrast near-infrared polarized reflectance images of demineralization on tooth buccal and occlusal surfaces at lambda = 1310-nm. Lasers Surg Med. 2009;41(3):208–13.

60. Fried WA, Chan KH, Fried D, Darling CL. High contrast reflectance imaging of simulated lesions on tooth occlusal surfaces at near-IR wavelengths. Lasers Surg Med. 2013;45:533–41.

61. Zhang L, Nelson LY, Seibel EJ. Spectrally enhanced imaging of occlusal surfaces and artificial shallow enamel erosions with a scanning fiber endoscope. J Biomed Opt. 2012;17(7):076019.

62. Spitzer D, ten Bosch JJ. The absorption and scattering of light in bovine and human dental enamel. Calcif Tiss Res. 1975;17:129–37.

63. Zijp JR, ten Bosch JJ, Groenhuis RA. HeNe laser light scattering by human dental enamel. J Dent Res. 1995;74:1891–8.

64. Simon JC, Chan KH, Darling CL, Fried D. Multispectral near-IR reflectance imaging of simulated early occlusal lesions: variation of lesion contrast with lesion depth and severity. Lasers Surg Med. 2014;46(3):203–15.

65. Alfano RR, Lam W, Zarrabi HJ, Alfano MA, Cordero J, Tata DB. Human teeth with and without caries studied by laser scattering, fluorescence and absorption spectroscopy. IEEE J Quant Electr. 1984;20:1512–5.

66. Bjelkhagen H, Sundstrom F. A clinically applicable laser luminescence for the early detection of dental caries. IEEE J Quant Electr. 1981;17:266–8.

67. Koenig K, Schneckenburger H, Hemmer J, Tromberg BJ, Steiner RW, Rudolf W. In-vivo fluorescence detection and imaging of porphyrin-producing bacteria in the human skin and in the oral cavity for diagnosis of acne vulgaris, caries, and squamous cell carcinoma. In: Advances in laser and light spectroscopy to diagnose cancer and other diseases. SPIE. vol. 2135; 1994. p. 129–138.

68. Shi XQ, Welander U, Angmar-Mansson B. Occlusal caries detection with Kavo DIAGNOdent and radiography: an in vitro comparison. Caries Res. 2000;34:151–8.

69. Lussi A, Hack A, Hug I, Heckenberger H, Megert B, Stich H. Detection of approximal caries with a new laser fluorescence device. Caries Res. 2006;40(2):97–103.

70. ten Bosch JJ. Summary of research of quantitative light fluorescence. In: Early detection of dental caries II. Indiana University. Vol. 4; 1999. p. 261–278.

71. Lakowicz JR. Principles of fluorecence spectroscopy. New York: Kluwer Academic; 1999.

72. Hafstroem-Bjoerkman U, de Josselin de Jong E, Oliveby A, Angmar-Mansson B. Comparison of laser fluorescence and longitudinal microradiography for quantitative assessment of *in vitro* enamel caries. Caries Res. 1992;26:241–7.

73. Ando M, Gonzalez-Cabezas C, Isaacs RL, Eckert AF, Stookey GK. Evaluation of several techniques for the detection of secondary caries adjacent to amalgam restorations. Caries Res. 2004;38:350–6.

74. de Josselin de Jong E, Sundstrom F, Westerling H, Tranaeus S, ten Bosch JJ, Angmar-Mansson B. A new method for in vivo quantification of changes in initial enamel caries with laser fluorescence. Caries Res. 1995;29(1):2–7.

75. Fontana M, Li Y, Dunipace AJ, Noblitt TW, Fischer G, Katz BP, Stookey GK. Measurement of enamel demineralization using microradiography and confocal microscopy. Caries Res. 1996;30:317–25.

76. Stookey GK. Quantitative light fluorescence: a technology for early monitoring of the caries process. Dent Clin North Am. 2005;49(4):753–70.

77. Amaechi BT, Podoleanu A, Higham SM, Jackson DA. Correlation of quantitative light-induced fluorescence and optical coherence tomography applied for detection and quantification of early dental caries. J Biomed Opt. 2003;8(4):642–7.

78. Ando M, Eckert GJ, Stookey GK, Zero DT. Effect of imaging geometry on evaluating natural white-spot lesions using quantitative light-induced fluorescence. Caries Res. 2004;38(1):39–44.

79. Ando M, Schemehorn BR, Eckert GJ, Zero DT, Stookey GK. Influence of enamel thickness on quantification of mineral loss in enamel using laser-induced fluorescence. Caries Res. 2003;37(1): 24–8.

80. al-Khateeb S, Oliveby A, de Josselin de Jong E, Angmar-Mansson B. Laser fluorescence quantification of remineralisation in situ of incipient enamel lesions: influence of fluoride supplements. Caries Res. 1997;31(2):132–40.

81. Tranaeus S, Al-Khateeb S, Bjorkman S, Twetman S, Angmar-Mansson B. Application of quantitative light-induced fluorescence to monitor incipient lesions in caries-active children. A comparative study of remineralisation by fluoride varnish and professional cleaning. Eur J Oral Sci. 2001;109(2):71–5.

82. al-Khateeb S, ten Cate JM, Angmar-Mansson B, de Josselin de Jong E, Sundstrom G, Exterkate RA, Oliveby A. Quantification of formation and remineralization of artificial enamel lesions with a new portable fluorescence device. Adv Dent Res. 1997;11(4):502–6.

83. Konig K, Schneckenburger H, Hibst R. Time-gated in vivo autofluorescence imaging of dental caries. Cell Mol Biol (Noisy-le-Grand). 1999;45(2):233–9.

84. Hall A, Girkin JM. A review of potential new diagnostic modalities for caries lesions. J Dent Res. 2004;83 Spec No C:C89–94.

85. Eggertsson H, Analoui M, MHvd V, Gonzalez-Cabezas C, Eckert GJ, Stookey GK. Detection of early interproximal caries in vitro using laser fluorescence, dye-enhanced laser fluorescence and direct visual examination. Caries Res. 1999;33:227–33.

86. Ando M, Hall AF, Eckert GJ, Schemehorn BR, Analoui M, Stookey GK. Relative ability of laser fluorescence techniques to quantitate early mineral loss in vitro. Caries Res. 1997;31(2):125–31.

87. Bouma BE, Tearney GJ. Handbook of optical coherence tomography. New York: Marcel Dekker; 2002.

88. Derickson D. Fiber optic test and measurement. Upper Saddle River: Prentice Hall; 1998.

89. Youngquist RC, Carr S, Davies DEN. Optical coherence-domain reflectometry. Appl Opt. 1987;12:158–60.

90. Huang D, Swanson EA, Lin CP, Schuman JS, Stinson WG, Chang W, Hee MR, Flotte T, Gregory K, Puliafito CA, Fujimoto JG. Optical coherence tomography. Science. 1991;254:1178–81.

91. Colston B, Everett M, Da Silva L, Otis L, Stroeve P, Nathel H. Imaging of hard and soft tissue structure in the oral cavity by optical coherence tomography. Appl Opt. 1998;37(19):3582–5.

92. Colston BW, Sathyam US, DaSilva LB, Everett MJ, Stroeve P. Dental OCT. Opt Express. 1998;3(3):230–8.

93. Feldchtein FI, Gelikonov GV, Gelikonov VM, Iksanov RR, Kuranov RV, Sergeev AM, Gladkova ND, Ourutina MN, Warren JA, Reitze DH. In vivo OCT imaging of hard and soft tissue of the oral cavity. Opt Express. 1998;3(3):239–51.

94. Rongguang L, Wong V, Marcus M, Burns P, McLaughlin P. Multimodal imaging system for dental caries detection. Proc SPIE Int Soc Opt Eng. 2008;6425:642502.
95. Madjarova VD, Yasuno Y, Makita S, Hori Y, Voeffray JB, Itoh M, Yatagai T, Tamura M, Nanbu T. Investigations of soft and hard tissues in oral cavity by spectral domain optical coherence tomography. In: Coherence domain optical methods and optical coherence tomography in biomedicine X. 2006;6079(1):60790N-60791-60797.
96. Seon YR, Jihoon N, Hae YC, Woo JC, Byeong HL, Gil-Ho Y. Realization of fiber-based OCT system with broadband photonic crystal fiber coupler. Proc SPIE Int Soc Opt Eng. 2006;6079(1):60791N-60791-60797.
97. Yamanari M, Makita S, Violeta DM, Yatagai T, Yasuno Y. Fiber-based polarization-sensitive Fourier domain optical coherence tomography using B-scan-oriented polarization modulation method. Opt Express. 2006;14(14):6502.
98. Furukawa H, Hiro-Oka H, Amano T, DongHak C, Miyazawa T, Yoshimura R, Shimizu K, Ohbayashi K. Reconstruction of three-dimensional structure of an extracted tooth by OFDR-OCT. In: Coherence domain optical methods and optical coherence tomography in biomedicine X. SPIE. vol. 6079; 2006. p. 60790T-60791-60797.
99. Amaechi BT, Higham SM, Podoleanu AG, Rodgers JA, Jackson DA. Use of optical coherence tomography for assessment of dental caries. J Oral Rehab. 2001;28(12):1092–3.
100. Sowa MG, Popescu DP, Friesen JR, Hewko MD, Choo-Smith LP. A comparison of methods using optical coherence tomography to detect demineralized regions in teeth. J Biophotonics. 2011;4(11–12):814–23.
101. Espigares J, Sadr A, Hamba H, Shimada Y, Otsuki M, Tagami J, Sumi Y. Assessment of natural enamel lesions with optical coherence tomography in comparison with microfocus x-ray computed tomography. J Med Imag. 2015;2(1):014001.
102. Baumgartner A, Hitzenberger CK, Dicht S, Sattmann H, Moritz A, Sperr W, Fercher AF. Optical coherence tomography for dental structures. In: Lasers in Dentistry IV. SPIE. vol. 3248; 1998. p. 130–136.
103. Baumgartner A, Dicht S, Hitzenberger CK, Sattmann H, Robi B, Moritz A, Sperr W, Fercher AF. Polarization-sensitive optical optical coherence tomography of dental structures. Caries Res. 2000;34:59–69.
104. Wang XJ, Zhang JY, Milner TE, JFd B, Zhang Y, Pashley DH, Nelson JS. Characterization of dentin and enamel by use of optical coherence tomography. Appl Opt. 1999;38(10):586–90.
105. Ko AC, Choo-Smith LP, Hewko M, Leonardi L, Sowa MG, Dong CC, Williams P, Cleghorn B. Ex vivo detection and characterization of early dental caries by optical coherence tomography and Raman spectroscopy. J Biomed Opt. 2005;10(3):031118.
106. Ko AC, Hewko M, Sowa MG, Dong CC, Cleghorn B, Choo-Smith LP. Early dental caries detection using a fibre-optic coupled polarization-resolved Raman spectroscopic system. Opt Express. 2008;16(9):6274–84.
107. Jones RS, Staninec M, Fried D. Imaging artificial caries under composite sealants and restorations. J Biomed Opt. 2004;9(6):1297–304.
108. Jones RS, Darling CL, Featherstone JDB, Fried D. Remineralization of in vitro dental caries assessed with polarization sensitive optical coherence tomography. J Biomed Opt. 2006;11(1):014016.
109. Jones RS, Darling CL, Featherstone JD, Fried D. Imaging artificial caries on the occlusal surfaces with polarization-sensitive optical coherence tomography. Caries Res. 2006;40(2):81–9.
110. Chan KH, Chan AC, Fried WA, Simon JC, Darling CL, Fried D. Use of 2D images of depth and integrated reflectivity to represent the severity of demineralization in cross-polarization optical coherence tomography. J Biophotonics. 2015;8(1–2):36–45.
111. Lee RC, Kang H, Darling CL, Fried D. Automated assessment of the remineralization of artificial enamel lesions with polarization-sensitive optical coherence tomography. Biomed Opt Express. 2014;5(9):2950–62.
112. Kang H, Darling CL, Fried D. Nondestructive monitoring of the repair of enamel artificial lesions by an acidic remineralization model using polarization-sensitive optical coherence tomography. Dent Mater. 2012;28(5):488–94.
113. Jones RS, Fried D. Remineralization of enamel caries can decrease optical reflectivity. J Dent Res. 2006;85(9):804–8.
114. Ngaotheppitak P, Darling CL, Fried D. Measurement of the severity of natural smooth surface (interproximal) caries lesions with polarization sensitive optical coherence tomography. Lasers Surg Med. 2005;37(1):78–88.
115. Lee RC, Darling CL, Fried D. Assessment of remineralization via measurement of dehydration rates with thermal and near-IR reflectance imaging. J Dent. 2015;43:36–45.
116. Le MH, Darling CL, Fried D. Automated analysis of lesion depth and integrated reflectivity in PS-OCT scans of tooth demineralization. Lasers Surg Med. 2010;42(1):62–8.
117. Kang H, Jiao JJ, Chulsung L, Le MH, Darling CL, Fried DL. Nondestructive assessment of early tooth demineralization using cross-polarization optical coherence tomography. IEEE J Sel Top Quantum Electron. 2010;16(4):870–6.
118. Makhija SK, Gilbert GH, Funkhouser E, Bader JD, Gordan VV, Rindal DB, Bauer M, Pihlstrom DJ, Qvist V, National Dental Practice-Based Research Network Collaborative Group. The prevalence of questionable occlusal caries: findings from the Dental Practice-Based Research Network. J Am Dent Assoc. 2012;143(12):1343–50.

119. Makhija SK, Gilbert GH, Funkhouser E, Bader JD, Gordan VV, Rindal DB, Pihlstrom DJ, Qvist V, National Dental PBRN Collaborative Group. Characteristics, detection methods and treatment of questionable occlusal carious lesions: findings from the national dental practice-based research network. Caries Res. 2014;48(3):200–7.

120. Makhija SK, Gilbert GH, Funkhouser E, Bader JD, Gordan VV, Rindal DB, Qvist V, Norrisgaard P, National Dental PBRN Collaborative Group. Twenty-month follow-up of occlusal caries lesions deemed questionable at baseline: findings from the National Dental Practice-Based Research Network. J Am Dent Assoc. 2014;145(11):1112–8.

121. Bader JD, Shugars DA. The evidence supporting alternative management strategies for early occlusal caries and suspected occlusal dentinal caries. J Evid Based Dent Pract. 2006;6(1):91–100.

122. Bader JD, Shugars DA, Bonito AJ. A systematic review of the performance of methods for identifying carious lesions. J Public Health Dent. 2002;62(4):201–13.

123. Douglas SM, Fried D, Darling CL. Imaging natural occlusal caries lesions with optical coherence tomograph. Proc SPIE Int Soc Opt Eng. 2010;7549:75490N.

124. Kang H, Darling CL, Fried D. Use of an optical clearing agent to enhance the visibility of subsurface structures and lesions from tooth occlusal surfaces. J Biomed Opt. 2016;21(8):081206.

125. Tuchin VV. Optical clearing of tissues and blood. Bellingham: SPIE; 2006.

126. Zhu D, Larin KV, Luo Q, Tuchin VV. Recent progress in tissue clearing. Laser Photonics Rev. 2013;7(5):732–57.

127. Jones RS, Fried D. The effect of high index liquids on PS-OCT imaging of dental caries. In: Lasers in Dentistry XI. SPIE. vol. 5687; 2005. p. 34–41.

128. Schmitt JM, Xiang SH, Yung KM. Speckle reduction techniques. In: Bouma BE, Tearney GJ, editors. Handbook of optical coherence tomography. 21st ed. New York: Marcel Dekker; 2002.

129. Marks DL, Ralston TS, Boppart SA. Data analysis and signal postprocessing for optical coherence tomography technology. In: Drexler W, Fujimoto JG, editors. Optical coherence tomography technology and applications. New York: Springer; 2008.

130. Rogowska J. Digital image processing techniques for speckle reduction, enhancement, and segmentation of optical coherence tomography (OCT) images. In: Brezinski M, editor. Optical coherence tomography: principles and applications. London: Elsevier; 2006.

131. Lee YK, Rhodes WT. Nonlinear image processing by a rotating kernel transformation. Opt Lett. 1990;15(23):1383–5.

132. Rogowska J, Brezinski ME. Evaluation of the adaptive speckle suppression filter for coronary optical coherence tomography imaging. IEEE Trans Med Imaging. 2000;19(12):1261–6.

133. Rogowska J, Brezinski ME. Image processing techniques for noise removal, enhancement and segmentation of cartilage OCT images. Phys Med Biol. 2002;47(4):641–55.

134. Amaechi BT, Podoleanu AG, Komarov G, Higham SM, Jackson DA. Quantification of root caries using optical coherence tomography and microradiography: a correlational study. Oral Health Prev Dent. 2004;2(4):377–82.

135. Lee C, Darling C, Fried D. Polarization sensitive optical coherence tomographic imaging of artificial demineralization on exposed surfaces of tooth roots. Dent Mat. 2009;25(6):721–8.

136. Manesh SK, Darling CL, Fried D. Nondestructive assessment of dentin demineralization using polarization-sensitive optical coherence tomography after exposure to fluoride and laser irradiation. J Biomed Mater Res B Appl Biomater. 2009;90(2):802–12.

137. Manesh SK, Darling CL, Fried D. Polarization-sensitive optical coherence tomography for the nondestructive assessment of the remineralization of dentin. J Biomed Opt. 2009;14(4):044002.

138. Manesh SK, Darling CL, Fried D. Nondestructive assessment of dentin demineralization using polarization sensitive optical coherence tomography. J Biomed Mater Res. 2009;90(2):802–12.

139. Wada I, Shimada Y, Ikeda M, Sadr A, Nakashima S, Tagami J, Sumi Y. Clinical assessment of non carious cervical lesion using swept-source optical coherence tomography. J Biophotonics. 2015;8(10):846–54.

140. Otis LL, Al-Sadhan RI, Meiers J, Redford-Badwal D. Identification of occlusal sealants using optical coherence tomography. J Clin Dent. 2000;14(1):7–10.

141. Stahl J, Kang H, Fried D. Imaging simulated secondary caries lesions with cross polarization OCT. Proc SPIE Int Soc Opt Eng. 2010;7549:754905.

142. Lammeier C, Li Y, Lunos S, Fok A, Rudney J, Jones RS. Influence of dental resin material composition on cross-polarization-optical coherence tomography imaging. J Biomed Opt. 2012;17(10):106002.

143. Lenton P, Rudney J, Chen R, Fok A, Aparicio C, Jones RS. Imaging in vivo secondary caries and ex vivo dental biofilms using cross-polarization optical coherence tomography. Dent Mater. 2012;28(7):792–800.

144. Holtzman JS, Osann K, Pharar J, Lee K, Ahn YC, Tucker T, Sabet S, Chen Z, Gukasyan R, Wilder-Smith P. Ability of optical coherence tomography to detect caries beneath commonly used dental sealants. Lasers Surg Med. 2010;42(8):752–9.

145. Tom H, Simon JC, Chan KH, Darling CL, Fried D. Near-infrared imaging of demineralization under sealants. J Biomed Opt. 2014;19(7):77003.

146. Louie T, Lee C, Hsu D, Hirasuna K, Manesh S, Staninec M, Darling CL, Fried D. Clinical assessment of early tooth demineralization using polarization sensitive optical coherence tomography. Lasers Surg Med. 2010;42:738–45.

147. Nee A, Chan K, Kang H, Staninec M, Darling CL, Fried D. Longitudinal monitoring of demineralization peripheral to orthodontic brackets using cross polarization optical coherence tomography. J Dent. 2014;42(5):547–55.

148. Chan KH, Tom H, Lee RC, Kang H, Simon JC, Staninec M, Darling CL, Pelzner RB, Fried D. Clinical monitoring of smooth surface enamel lesions using CP-OCT during nonsurgical intervention. Lasers Surg Med. 2016;48(10):915–23.

149. Hale GM, Querry MR. Optical constants of water in the 200-nm to 200-μm wavelength region. Appl Opt. 1973;12:555–63.

150. Koenig K, Schneckenburger H. Laser-induced Autofluorescence for Medical Diagnosis. J Fluorescence 1993; 4(1):17–40.

151. Zhang L, Kim AS, Ridge JS, Nelson LY, Berg JH, Seibel EJ. Trimodal detection of early childhood caries using laser light scanning and fluorescence spectroscopy: clinical prototype. J Biomed Opt. 2013;18(11):111412.

Endodontics and Pulpal Diagnosis

Jan M. O'Dell

Introduction

When a patient presents to a healthcare provider, it is often with the expectation that the practitioner will "fix what ails" the patient. The practitioner must develop a plan of treatment based on an accurate diagnosis. This treatment can be for a variety of reasons. Most often, the goal of treatment is to eliminate the disease process which the patient has and to provide a cure. Or treatment may be geared to treat chronic conditions or maintain some discrete level of health, for example, with hypertension. Or treatment may be initiated to provide only palliative care. In any case, an accurate diagnosis is essential. Without an accurate diagnosis, any proposed treatment may result in an adverse outcome for the patient.

In 1963, Robinson defined diagnosis as the "identification of the nature of an illness or other problem by examination of the symptoms" [1]. This is most frequently accomplished by incorporating several different but complementary methods of data collection to determine if there is any deviation from normal. Among the most useful items contributing to an accurate diagnosis are the patient's chief complaint, a review of both the patient's medical and dental history, and the performance of diagnostic tests.

It is paramount to remember that treatment cannot be initiated unless and until a preliminary or differential diagnosis has been determined. The patient must be fully informed about the proposed treatment, alternatives to proposed treatment, and consequences of no treatment. Included in this discussion between the patient and clinician are the potential risks and the expected outcome of treatment. The patient must fully understand and have an opportunity to ask questions regarding treatment.

Because patients often seek care only when they are in pain, the clinician should always proceed in a thorough manner and not skip steps in an attempt to quickly relieve the patients' pain.

Medical History

The importance of obtaining a complete and accurate medical history cannot be overstated. With patients living longer and often taking multiple medications, it is necessary to have a thorough understanding of the conditions and medications that may alert the clinician to the need for consulting with the patient's physician before starting treatment. The first step in obtaining a medical history is to have the patient(s), or care giver(s), complete a health history form. Every question should be answered, and any condition that is identified should elicit further investigation. There are many medical conditions that have oral

J. M. O'Dell (✉)
Department of Endodontics, UTHSC College of Dentistry, Memphis, TN, USA
e-mail: jodell10@uthsc.edu

© Springer Nature Switzerland AG 2020
P. Wilder-Smith, J. Ajdaharian (eds.), *Oral Diagnosis*, https://doi.org/10.1007/978-3-030-19250-1_2

implications, and some non-odontogenic conditions may mimic dental pain. Among the most common is a maxillary sinusitis that may present as a toothache in the maxillary posterior quadrant. Or the patient(s) may insist that a particular tooth is causing pain when in fact the patients are suffering from trigeminal neuralgia [2]. It is important to remember that often patients have a very different idea of what is to be included. For example, the patients may only mark "yes" to a question regarding illness if they have been hospitalized, or they may not include medications taken except those drugs prescribed by a physician. There are several sources available to obtain generic health history forms, or they may be developed by the practitioner with areas of particular interest emphasized. In any event, the health history must be reviewed at every appointment, and vital signs recorded (Fig. 1). If, after review of the medical history, it is determined that a medical consultation is warranted, documentation should include the physician, date, and rea-

son for the consultation (Fig. 2), and the response should be entered into the patient's records. Furthermore, it will be necessary to have the patient(s) sign a consent for treatment and the release of such protected information (see Fig. 2).

Dental History

There are two components to the dental history. First is a general history, which should focus on previous treatment as well as any problems the patient may have encountered. Then, the history of the present illness should be taken. This is most often centered around the patient's chief complaint. The chief complaint should be recorded verbatim and is the reason the patient is seeking treatment. The patient is asked the nature and severity of the problem. This is easily accomplished by providing the patient with a preprinted form (Fig. 3). Included on this form should be simple "yes" or "no" questions, as well

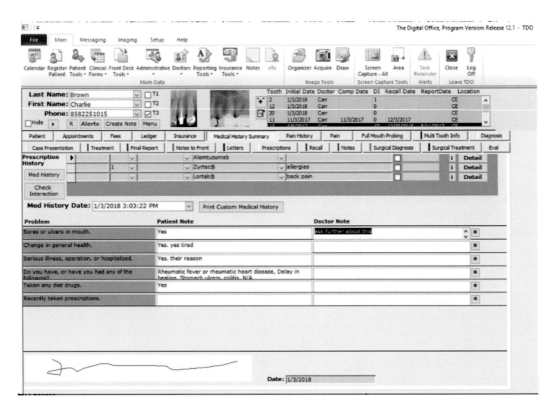

Fig. 1 Health history form. (Courtesy of Dr. G. Carr, TDO)

The
Dental SPECIALISTS

MEDICAL/CONSULTATION REQUEST

Patient Name _____ DOB _____ Patient # _____

Home Phone _____ Work Phone _____

CONSULTATION

Dr. _____Telephone _____

Address _____

HISTORY AND PHYSICAL FINDINGS

_____

_____

_____

SERVICES DESIRED

_____

_____

_____

Doctor Signature _____ Patient Signature _____ Date _____

(If applicable)

PHYSICAN'S RESPONSE

_____

_____

_____

_____

_____

_____

_____

Signature _____ Date _____

** PLEASE RETURN RESPONSE TO THE PRACTICE _____

_____

_____

Attn: Dr. _____

TDS-16082

Fig. 2 Medical consultation form. (Courtesy of Dr. A. Law, The Dental Specialists)

as open-ended questions to allow the patient to explain or characterize and quantify the symptoms. There should be questions regarding recent dental procedures, trauma, and what if anything elicits or relieves the pain. It is also important to record if the patient has taken any analgesic that may alter diagnostic testing results.

Patient Examination

The patient examination should start the moment the patient arrives at the dental office. Included in this generalized physical exam should be an evaluation of the patient's posture and gait, exposed skin surfaces, vital signs, mental acuity, and the ability to communicate. Often the patient who presents with acute pain has visible signs of swelling, redness, lack of sleep, etc., which may contribute to inaccurate information. Once the patient is seated, evaluation of both extraoral and intraoral structures should be accomplished to determine if there are any abnormalities (Fig. 4a). If any lesion is identified, the location, size, color, and shape should be recorded and followed to resolution. Also, an oral cancer screening should always be performed and findings recorded (Fig. 4b).

SADDLEBACK VALLEY ENDODONTICS

Pain History

---

1. Have you experienced pain in this tooth any time in the past?
    ☐ Yes   ☐ No (If you are not in pain now and have never been in pain with this tooth, go directly to question #17).

2. Are you in pain now?
    ☐ Yes   ☐ No

3. If you are in pain now, how long have you been in pain?
    ☐ 1 day   ☐ 2 days   ☐ 3 days   ☐ 4 day   ☐ 5 days
    ☐ 6 days   ☐ 1 week   ☐ 2 weeks   ☐ 3 week   ☐ > 3 weeks

4. Did this pain either keep you awake or awaken you last night?
    ☐ Yes   ☐ Yes, and I have been up all night in pain
    ☐ Yes   ☐ No, but it has before

5. Can you locate the tooth that is causing the pain?
    ☐ Yes   ☐ No   ☐ Not Sure   ☐ There may be more than one tooth

6. Does the pain radiate to other parts of your jaw or down your neck and shoulders?
    ☐ Yes   ☐ No   ☐ No, but it has in the past

7. Is the pain spontaneous or does it always require some stimulus to become painful?
    ☐ I have spontaneous pain   ☐ It always takes some stimulus to make it hurt
    ☐ I don't have spontaneous pain now, but I have in the past with this tooth

8. Do you feel swollen now?
             ☐ Yes   ☐ No
    Has there been a history of prior swelling?
             ☐ Yes   ☐ No
    Are you running a fever?
             ☐ Yes   ☐ No

9. How would you rate the severity of your pain today? (as a number and as a description, 10 being unbearable, 1 being very slight)?
    ☐ 1   ☐ 2   ☐ 3   ☐ 4   ☐ 5   ☐ 6   ☐ 7   ☐ 8   ☐ 9   ☐ 10

10. Do you have lingering pain?
    ☐ Yes   ☐ No   ☐ No, but I have in the past

11. Please check the frequency and nature of the pain that most accurately describes your discomfort.
    ☐ Sharp   ☐ Dull   ☐ Radiating
    ☐ Throbbing ☐ Migrating   ☐ Constant
    ☐ Aching   ☐ Intermittent ☐ Momentary
    ☐ Gnawing   ☐ Variable   ☐ Enlarging to other areas
    ☐ Shooting   ☐ Tingling   ☐ Itching
    ☐ Yes   ☐ Only when chewing or biting

Fig. 3 Dental history form. (Courtesy of Dr. S. McNicholas, Saddleback Valley Endodontists)

12. Is the tooth sensitive to temperature?
☐ No, but there is a history of temperature sensitivity in the past
☐ More to hot than cold   ☐ Equally to hot and cold
☐ Neither   ☐ Not sure   ☐ More sensitive to cold than hot

13. What relieves the pain?
☐ Nothing   ☐ Cold   ☐ Hot   ☐ Massage   ☐ Vicodin
☐ Non-biting   ☐ Aspirin   ☐ NSAIDS   ☐ Codeine   ☐ Advil / Aleve
☐ Antibiotics   ☐ Other   ☐ Darvon / Darvocet   ☐ Tylenol

14. If you don't touch the tooth or bite on it, does it still hurt?
☐ Yes   ☐ No   ☐ Sometimes ☐ Only if I bite a certain way
☐ Not now, but it has in the past

15. What increases the pain?
☐ Touching   ☐ Biting   ☐ Cold   ☐ Hot   ☐ Eating   ☐ Cold air
☐ Lying down   ☐ Pressing on gum   ☐ Flossing   ☐ Nothing   ☐ Sweets

16. What is the course of pain?
☐ Increasing   ☐ Decreasing   ☐ Constant   ☐ Variable   ☐ None now

17. Has there been any recent restorative work done on this area?
☐ Yes   ☐ No   ☐ Not sure

18. Prior to this appointment has endodontic treatment been started by any doctor?
☐ Yes   ☐ No   ☐ Unknown

19. Have you had recent periodontal (gum) surgery or a recent tooth cleaning?
☐ Yes   ☐ No

20. Have you ever had any endodontic surgery (apico) done on this tooth?
☐ Yes   ☐ No   ☐ Unknown

21. Are you numb now (been given anesthesia earlier today)?
☐ Yes   ☐ No   ☐ Slightly   ☐ Not sure

22. Have you taken any antibiotics for this problem?
☐ No   ☐ Today   ☐ Last 2 days   ☐ Last 3 days
☐ Last 4 days   ☐ Last week   ☐ Last month   ☐ Other

22. Have you taken any pain medication for this problem?
☐ No   ☐ Today   ☐ Last night
☐ Last 2 days   ☐ Last 3 days   ☐ Last 4 days
☐ Last 5 days   ☐ Last 6 days   ☐ Various times

23. Did you explicitly request this referral?
☐ Yes   ☐ No

24. Did your doctor recommend this referral?
☐ Yes   ☐ No

Fig. 3 (continued)

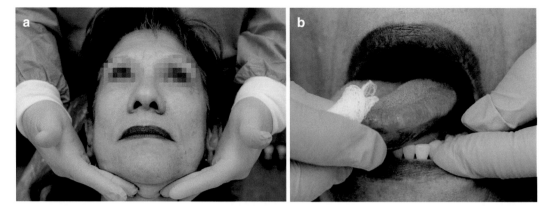

Fig. 4 Patient examination. (**a**) Extraoral exam. (**b**) Oral cancer screening

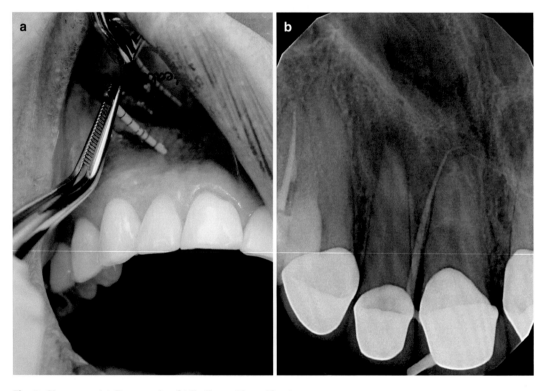

Fig. 5 Sinus tract. (**a**) Gutta percha. (**b**) Radiographic verification

After review of the general dental history and chief complaint, the clinician may have a good idea of what area or tooth is contributing to the patient's pain. However, a complete exam should still be performed to confirm the patient's information. The intraoral exam should include a general assessment of oral soft tissues, hard tissues, and dentition. The generalized periodontal condition, carious lesions, enamel frac-tures, discolored teeth, as well as missing and restored dentition should all be noted. If a soft tissue lesion is discovered, with a sinus tract, it should be traced with gutta percha and a radio-graph taken to confirm the origin of the lesion (Fig. 5).

Once a general assessment of the patient's dentition is completed, it is time to concentrate on diagnostic tests with the goal of confirming the clinician's preliminary determination of pulpal status, which in turn will provide the basis for treatment.

Traditional Clinical Tests to Assess Pulpal Status

Chambers [3] stated that the determination of the pulp status is critical to an accurate diagnosis. He added that "the ideal pulp test should provide a simple, objective, standardized reproducible and inexpensive method of assessing the exact condition of the pulp tissue at any given time." Ehrmann [4] recommends evaluating the pulp status before restorative procedures. This is important because the patient may not be experiencing pain even though the tooth is not responding to vitality tests. Vitality may be absent long before radiographic signs are apparent, or the patient is symptomatic. Traditionally, the primary use of vitality tests has been as an aid in the diagnosis of pain and as an adjunct to the radiographic investigation. Additional uses have been suggested by Mumford and Bjorn [5] and include posttraumatic evaluation, determination of pulp vitality following previous pulp therapy or assessment of teeth that have been heavily restored. It has also been suggested

that a pulpal response can be used to determine if a tooth is exhibiting profound pulpal anesthesia.

Alghaithy et al. [6] describes the use of a "reference standard" which does not necessarily identify the target condition with 100% accuracy. A reference standard enables the measurement of sensitivity, specificity, and accuracy. The gold standard is the best available method against which the performance of other diagnostic or index tests is evaluated. The gold standard for the determination of pulp status is histopathology. Unfortunately this is not possible in clinical settings. Most current methods employed by clinicians depend on the sensory response of the pulp rather than pulpal blood flow, even though the latter provides a more predictable assessment of vitality [7, 8]. Banes and Hammond [9] discussed the work by Johnson and Hinds demonstrating that a test may elicit a negative response even though there may still be vital pulp tissue if the test is only able to gain information on a neural level.

When performing any test, it is advisable to test at a minimum one tooth mesial and distal, and possibly the opposing or contralateral tooth to provide a control or baseline reading.

Terms for both pulpal (Table 1) and periapical diagnosis (Table 2) are described and represent the most current descriptions [10].

Table 1 Clinical classification of pulpal diagnosis

Terminology	Clinical findings	Radiographic findings	Treatment
Normal pulp	Symptom-free and normally responsive to pulp testing	Radiographic findings show no evidence of resorption or decay	No endodontic treatment needed
Reversible pulpitis	Based on subjective and objective findings. Stimulation is uncomfortable but reverses quickly upon removal. Inflamed pulp normally capable of healing	Radiographic findings may disclose caries or defective restorations	Conservative removal of irritant will normally resolve symptoms
Symptomatic irreversible pulpitis	Based on subjective and objective findings indicating the vital inflamed pulp is incapable of healing. Intermittent or spontaneous pain. Exposure to stimuli elicits heightened and/or prolonged response. Pain may be sharp, dull, localized, diffuse, or referred	Early stages fail to show any change in radiographic appearance. In advanced cases, there may be a thickening of the periodontal ligament radiographically. There may be deep restoration, caries, pulp exposure, direct, or indirect pulp therapy	Endodontic treatment. If left untreated, the pulp will eventually become necrotic

(continued)

Table 1 (continued)

Terminology	Clinical findings	Radiographic findings	Treatment
Asymptomatic irreversible pulpitis	Based on subjective and objective findings indicating that the vital inflamed pulp is incapable of healing. Patient does not complain of pain. Clinical and/or radiographic evidence of caries extending into the pulp	Radiographically, there is evidence of caries extending into the pulp	Endodontic treatment. If left untreated, tooth may become symptomatic, and pulp will become necrotic
Pulp necrosis	Based on subjective and objective findings indicating that the pulp is nonresponsive to pulp testing. It follows irreversible pulpitis and attempts to describe the histologic status of the pulp. Tooth will typically become symptom free until there is an extension of the disease process into the periradicular tissue. Tooth is normally nonresponsive to cold or electric stimulation, but may respond to heat stimuli. Pulp necrosis may be partial or complete resulting in confusing responses to testing	Radiographic changes may include a thickening of the periodontal ligament space or the appearance of a periapical radiolucent lesion	Endodontic treatment
Previously treated (accurate pretreatment diagnosis may not be possible)	Based on objective findings indicating the tooth has been endodontically treated and the canals are obturated with a medicament or filling material. Patient may or may not present with signs or symptoms	May or may not show radiographic evidence of thickened periodontal ligament space or appearance of a periapical radiolucent lesion. There is evidence of an intracanal medicament or canal obturation with a filling material	If patient is asymptomatic and there are no clinical or radiographic signs or symptoms of disease, no treatment may be indicated. If patient exhibits clinical or radiographic signs or symptoms, the tooth will require additional nonsurgical or surgical endodontic procedures to retain the tooth
Previously initiated therapy (accurate pretreatment diagnosis may not be possible)	Based on objectives findings that a tooth has been previously treated by partial endodontic therapy such as a pulpotomy or pulpectomy. This is often an emergency procedure, but may include vital pulp therapy, treatment of traumatic injury, apexification or apexogenesis	May or may not show radiographic evidence of thickened periodontal ligament space or appearance of a periapical radiolucent lesion. There may be evidence of an intracanal medicament but will not show evidence of canal obturation	Endodontic treatment

Terms are consistent with those of the AAE Glossary of Terms, 9th ed., 2016

Table 2 Clinical classification of periapical diagnosis

Terminology	Clinical findings	Radiographic findings
Normal apical tissues	Patient is asymptomatic and the tooth responds normally to percussion and palpation	Radiograph reveals an intact lamina dura and periodontal ligament space around all root apices
Symptomatic apical periodontitis	Inflammation, usually of the apical periodontium producing clinical symptoms including a painful response to biting, percussion, or palpation. Tooth may or may not respond to pulp vitality tests	Tooth will typically exhibit at least a widened periodontal ligament space. May or may not show an apical radiolucency associated with one or all of the roots
Asymptomatic apical periodontitis	Inflammation and destruction of the apical periodontium of pulpal origin; however, the patient is usually symptom free. Tooth typically will not respond to vitality tests	There is normally an apical radiolucent area around one or more of the roots
Acute apical abscess	An inflammatory reaction to pulpal infection and necrosis. Patient may experience one or more of the following symptoms: rapid onset, spontaneous pain, tenderness to pressure, pus formation, and swelling. Acute pain on biting, percussion, and palpation. There is no response to any pulp vitality tests. May exhibit varying degrees of mobility. In addition, patient may exhibit lymph involvement, fever, and swelling	Will vary from a widened periodontal ligament space to an apical radiolucency
Chronic apical abscess	Chronic inflammatory reaction to pulpal infection and necrosis. There is often no discomfort or a gradual onset of pain. There may be an associated sinus tract with intermittent discharge of pus. Tooth is nonresponsive to pulp vitality tests	Radiographically the tooth will exhibit a periapical radiolucency around one or more root apices

Terms are consistent with those of the AAE Glossary of Terms, 9th ed., 2016

Periodontal Examination

Mobility can be used to determine if the periodontal attachment apparatus is compromised. Berman and Rotstein [11] have suggested several possible reasons for tooth mobility. Among them are all types of trauma, periodontal disease, root fractures, or an extension of pulpal disease that has extended into the periodontal ligament. If the causative factors can be corrected, the mobility may improve. To perform a mobility test, use the flat ends of two instruments such as the mirror handle or perio-probe and place one end on the buccal surface while the other is on the lingual (Fig. 6). Pressure is then applied in a buccal–lingual direction and given a score of 1–3 according to O'Leary [12].

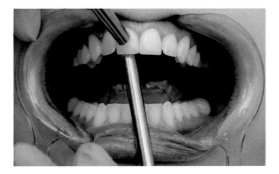

Fig. 6 Mobility test

Periodontal probing should also be measured and recorded (Fig. 7a, b). A solid knowledge of root morphology is essential when probing interproximal and furcation areas. In general, a probing that spreads across a tooth is considered broad and suggests a periodontal origin. However, if the probing is isolated and deep, it is suggestive of a defect of endodontic origin. It is imperative that a pulpal diagnosis is included when deciding on the appropriate treatment and prognosis. For example, the probing may be indicative of a vertical root fracture, in which case the long-term prognosis may be considered poor or hopeless. On the other hand, it may be endodontic in origin with a periodontal component, which may resolve with appropriate treatment. If a vertical root fracture is suspected, it may be necessary to anesthetize the area to "sneak" into the defect, which often will then extend to the apex of the root (Fig. 7c).

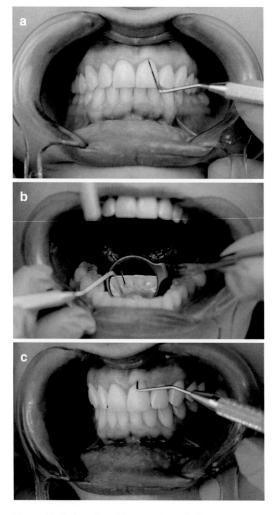

Fig. 7 Periodontal probing. (**a**) Buccal. (**b**) Lingual. (**c**) Vertical root fracture

Mechanical Tests

The primary mechanical tests include palpation, percussion, transillumination, bite testing, test cavities, isolated anesthesia, and electric pulp testing. These tests, while limited in their usefulness in determining the actual state of pulpal health, may provide valuable information in applicable situations.

Palpation

While not necessarily considered a test of pulpal vitality, this test is often the first test performed by the clinician. Its advantage lies in the ease by which it can be performed. There is no equipment required, it only takes a minute or two to complete, and apprehensive patients usually tolerate the test well. It can be performed with very little digital pressure which can be repeated with increasing pressure until a response is elicited. The purpose is to detect areas of soft tissue swelling or bony expansion when compared to adjacent and contralateral areas.

Palpation is performed by the application of gentle finger apical pressure (Fig. 8a) and asking the patient to respond to any area of discomfort. It is also possible to perform this test using a cotton tip applicator (Fig. 8b). However, the amount of pressure applied is not as consistent and patients will often provide a false-positive response to pressure upon palpation with the cotton tip applicator. It is therefore recommended to use increasing digital pressure. A positive response may suggest an active inflammatory response of the periapical tissue. Unfortunately, this test is, however, not conclusive for pain of endodontic origin.

Percussion

Percussion is very valuable as an indirect measure of pulpal involvement. Kulilid [13] has described three clinical situations that may present with a positive response to percussion. The most frequent and easiest to treat is following the recent placement of a restoration that is high in

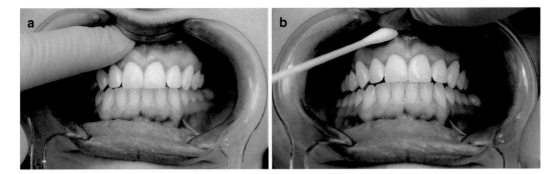

Fig. 8 Palpation. (**a**) Digital. (**b**) Cotton tip applicator

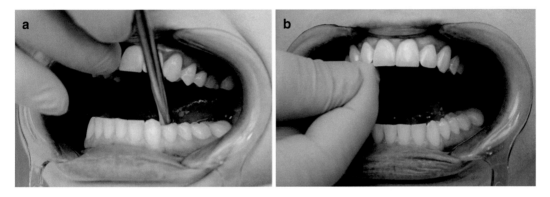

Fig. 9 Percussion. (**a**) Instrument. (**b**) Digital pressure

occlusion. Often the patient will indicate that a restoration was recently placed and the symptoms did not appear until after the appointment. To relieve symptoms, mark the patient's occlusion. Then with no anesthesia, if possible, perform any adjustment necessary until the patient is comfortable biting and moving through excursive movements. Often the patient will experience immediate relief. However, occasionally the nerve has undergone significant trauma and the patient will experience immediate relief but will return within a few days with the same complaint. At this point, the clinician must decide if endodontic intervention is appropriate. The second case is when the pulp has become necrotic, and a periapical lesion has developed. The patient, in this case, will often state that the tooth feels high but can be compressed back into the socket because it feels "mushy." Early sensitivity to percussion may not be associated with any radiographic evidence of periapical pathology; however, there is often the presence of large existing restorations on the tooth in question. With further testing, the tooth will typically be non-responsive to other routine diagnostic tests. Finally, it may also be possible to determine if a tooth has a coronal fracture. In this case, the tooth may be sensitive to percussion while also responding to thermal stimuli.

Anxiety by the patient may be decreased or eliminated by a simple explanation to the patient of what to expect. Initially, using the mirror handle or other similar instrument, gently tap on several control teeth from the occlusal or incisal surface before testing the suspect tooth (Fig. 9a). When it is not possible to isolate a particular tooth based on an abnormal response, wait for 3–4 minutes and retest with increasing the pressure. It may also be necessary to repeat this test tapping from the buccal or facial and lingual surfaces. An alternative to tapping with an instrument has been suggested by Kulilid [13]. He

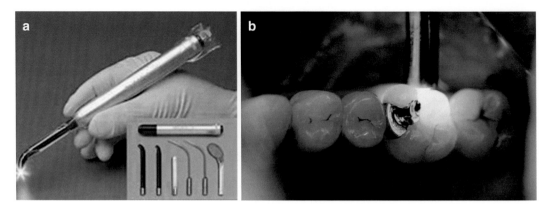

Fig. 10 Fiber-optic illumination. (**a**) Instrumentation. (**b**) Clinical use

recommends using digital compression of the tooth into the socket until the patient can discriminate between teeth being tested (Fig. 9b).

Percussion testing is considered one of the oldest diagnostic tools available. It is very easy to accomplish and provides good information regarding the inflammation of the periodontal ligament, indirectly implicating the health of the pulp. However, it is difficult to consistently reproduce the amount of pressure being used, perhaps leading to both false-positive and false-negative results. Many necrotic teeth may respond normally to percussion tests, especially if the disease process has not affected the periodontal ligament. To control this variable, Weisman [14] reports on the development and use of a calibrated percussion instrument. The instrument has a spring-loaded piston allowing the clinician to set the instrument at one of six equal preset graduated positions. Unfortunately, this instrument has not proven to provide information that is superior to that obtained by the quick and easy-to-use manual method.

Transillumination

Transillumination involves the passage of light through hard or soft tissue. It is based on the principle that as light passes through the interface between two structures or tissues of different refractive indices, it bends, producing areas with varying appearances of brightness. Transillumination of teeth can be a valuable addition to routine diagnostic tests, particularly when symptoms are vague or not consistent. Hill suggests transillumination can be useful for determining the vitality of a tooth when combined with thermal tests [15]. Friedman and Marcus [16] found transillumination to be useful in the detection of caries or calculus; however, it is more beneficial in the identification of coronal fractures and has been shown to be of value in teeth that have undergone traumatic injuries. While any small direct light source will accomplish transillumination, it is most frequently performed with a fiber-optic light source such as the Microlux™ (AdDent, Danbury, CT) (Fig. 10a). This allows cold, high-intensity light to be used with ease and flexibility.

During transillumination, isolation with a rubber dam will provide the best result. The operatory light should be turned off. The fiber-optic light source is then placed on the surface of the tooth in question (Fig. 10b). When evaluating a posterior tooth, it is best to confirm findings by placing the light on both the buccal and lingual surface. If there is a cusp fracture or a marginal ridge fracture, the side of the tooth with the light source will be illuminated leaving the tooth structure past the fracture darker in appearance. Identification of factures with this method is easy and accurate, but it fails to provide any information on the extent of the fracture or the status of the pulp. Further investigation with additional diagnostic tests should be performed to assess the status of the pulp. A bite test will often confirm the initial diagnosis of a coronal or root fracture.

Occasionally, the heavily restored tooth may result in difficulty identifying a crack. In this situation, it may be helpful to place a small amount of methylene blue dye on the tooth, waiting a few minutes then rinsing and applying a gentle stream of air to dry the tooth prior to observation with the fiber-optic light source. The dye will penetrate the fracture and make it more visible. It is important to be sensitive to the patient's complaint as the application of water and/or air may cause discomfort in the patient.

In addition to fracture detection, transillumination can be useful following trauma as the tooth may exhibit a subtle change in color. A healthy tooth will appear white with a yellow or pink hue. Following trauma and subsequent damage to the pulp, the tooth may appear brown, gray, or a darker shade of yellow.

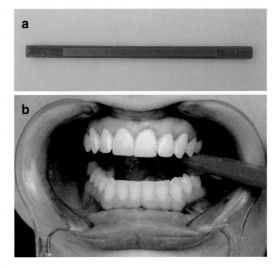

Fig. 11 Bite tests. (**a**) Instrumentation. (**b**) Clinical use

Bite Test

A patient may present with a complaint of pain with biting or chewing. Frequently, the patient will add that the pain is sporadic and difficult to localize. Adding a bite test to the transillumination test can often confirm the presence of a fracture. If the pulp has suffered enough damage, it may affect the periodontal ligament, resulting in an inflammatory response. There have been a variety of devices used in the past that are easy and convenient for the practitioner to use. These include a cotton tip applicator, cotton roll, orangewood sticks, etc. More recently, several devices have been developed specifically for testing sensitivity to biting. Tooth Slooth® (Professional Results, Laguna Niguel, CA) is but one example (Fig. 11a). It is shaped like a double-ended toothbrush with one end having a divot and the other having a raised area. In this manner, the clinician can test each cusp independently as well as apply pressure directly in an occlusal apical direction. To reproduce the patient's chief complaint, patients are instructed to bite firmly and

then release quickly, making note as to whether the pain elicited is on biting pressure or on release (Fig. 11b). If it is determined that the tooth has a fracture but responds normally to other diagnostic tests, the patient may elect to have a full coverage restoration placed. The patient should be advised that the tooth may require endodontic therapy in the future.

Test Cavity

Even after a thorough exam and completion of diagnostic tests, it may not be possible for the clinician to identify the source of the patient's pain. In these circumstances, it has been suggested that a test cavity be performed on the tooth suspected of causing the pain. Teeth most frequently subject to a test cavity are those with full coverage restorations and subgingival margins and teeth that have extensive calcification.

The patient is informed of the proposed procedure and must understand that it is an irreversible procedure performed without anesthesia. A small class one preparation is made using a high speed and small round bur with air and water. If the patient feels a painful sensation, the procedure is stopped, and the tooth is restored [17]. It is presumed that the tooth still has some viable nerve tissue remaining. Ehrmann, however, recommends the use of a slow-speed so the cavity can be kept shallow, extending only into the dentine [4]. Jafarzadeh [8] states that a test cavity is unlikely to provide definitive information and suggests that the diagnosis will depend on the skill and experience of the clinician. He concludes his review stating "test cavities are not justified in modern endodontic or dental practice and in the best interests of the patient."

Isolated Anesthesia

Similar to the test cavity, the application of isolated anesthesia is rarely used. However, it can be very helpful in determining the location of the offending tooth or if the pain is of odontogenic origin. This test is only useful when the patient presents with pain at the time of examination. For example, a patient may complain of pain in the mandible. If diagnostic tests suggest that all teeth in the area are vital, and if the pain remains following the administration of anesthetic, it may be cardiac in origin, and a referral to a physician is indicated. Similarly, a patient may complain of radiating pain in the maxillary arch and cheek. It may be possible to rule out a tooth as the source of pain and recommend evaluation for acute sinusitis, or perhaps neuralgia [18].

Electric Pulp Testing (EPT)

The use of electricity to determine tooth vitality originated in the late 1800s. While Marshall has been credited with describing the application of electricity to evaluate tooth health in 1891, Jafarzadeh places the earliest application of electrical current to stimulate pulp tissue in the 1878 Treatise on Dental Caries by Magitot [8]. EPT works by direct stimulation of sensory nerves in the pulp tissue. The nerves stimulated with the electric current are the A-delta nociceptors, and the result is often reported as a tingling or painful response by the patient. Most modern EPT systems are monopolar with a single electrode. With monopolar instruments, the current flows through all tissues between the electrodes. However, on occasion the EPT can produce a false-positive result as there may be excitation of nerves other than those of the pulp. Nahri [19] found that the threshold for pulp tissue is lower than for non-pulp tissue, so that activation of non-pulp tissue is unlikely. Newer models such as the Vitality Scanner™ (Kerr Dental, Orange, CA) (Fig. 12a) are frequently battery powered and have a power output that increases automatically to avoid a full charge on the initial application. Seltzer et al. [20, 21] found results are most accurate when no response is obtained, irrespective of the current applied. The lack of response is indicative of a necrotic pulp. A study by Peterson et al. [22] found the sensitivity (identification of teeth with disease) was 72%, compared to 83% for cold and 86% for heat. Specificity (identification of teeth without disease) revealed that 93% of teeth with a healthy pulp were correctly identified with thermal tests, but only 41% of teeth were correctly identified with electric testing. Their conclusion was electric testing had an accuracy of 71% compared to 86% with cold and 81% with heat.

Techniques for obtaining the most accurate results with the EPT will depend on several factors such as isolation, the speed which the current is applied, restorations and placement of the probe. As with other diagnostic procedures, it is best to begin testing on an adjacent tooth to obtain baseline healthy vales. The teeth being evaluated should be isolated with cotton rolls or with a rubber dam. Myers [23] found that if there are teeth with contacting amalgam restorations, the current can travel between them which could result in false readings. Following isolation, the teeth are then dried and the electrode placed on either the incisal or buccal surface of the tooth with a conducting medium (Fig. 12b). Since clinicians now routinely wear gloves, in order to complete the circuit, the patient should be instructed to hold the end of the probe [24]. The current is then gradually increased until the patient reports a "tingling" sensation. If the instrument reaches the maximum reading without eliciting any response it is presumed that the tooth being tested is necrotic. Practitioners should consider the EPT to be an "all or none" test. Michaelson et al. [25] evaluated different interface media,

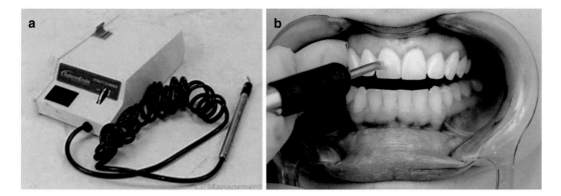

Fig. 12 Electric pulp testing. (**a**) Instrumentation. (**b**) Clinical use

including toothpaste, water, and EKG paste. Each material was tested on the facial and lingual surfaces, and the results showed no appreciable difference between the materials as long as the material was either water or petroleum-based. Because of its ease and availability, most clinicians use toothpaste as a conducting medium. It is imperative that the probe makes contact with the tooth, not with metallic or other restorations. A study by Bender et al. [26] found that when the probe was placed in the incisal region in an area of exposed dentin there was a significant decrease in the threshold response compared to the cervical and middle third. Contrary results were found in a study by Jacobson. In their laboratory study, the middle third of the incisor and the occlusal third of the premolars elicited the least resistance [27]. Multiple readings should be taken, and the results averaged to ensure that if there was a lack of response, it was not due to faulty positioning of the probe.

EPT has the advantage of providing better results in teeth with much secondary dentin where thermal tests have not produced adequate results [4]. Fuss et al. [28] found that ETP was more dependable than ethyl chloride or ice, which was in agreement with Ehrmann's results.

Concern regarding the use of electric tests in patients with cardiac pacemakers was first studied by Woolley, Woodworth, and Dobbs [29] using a canine model. Their results suggested that the magnitude of currents used could affect the pacemaker function and cautioned clinicians against using these devices in patients with cardiac pacemakers. Contrary to the work of Woolley et al. in

2006, Wilson et al. [30] concurred with the findings of Simon, stating that there was no effect on implanted cardiac pacemakers with either the electric pulp testers or electronic apex locators [31]. However, consulting the patient's physician is still recommended if there is any question concerning the patient's cardiac condition.

In addition to the concerns above, the electric pulp tester can be awkward to use, especially in a crowded dentition, a heavily restored dentition, or in the patient undergoing orthodontic treatment. Fulling and Andreasen [32] reported a higher current threshold for teeth with immature apices. Hyman and Cohen [33] also found that teeth with open apices usually gave little or no response. Until innervation is complete (4–5 years after teeth have been in function), electric testing is not a reliable means of determining tooth vitality [8].

Thermal Tests

Thermal testing is one of the oldest and most commonly used diagnostic tests. It involves either the application of a cooling agent to lower the tooth temperature or applying heat to raise the temperature of the tooth, both in an attempt to elicit a response from the patient. However, like the electric pulp tests, there is only a symptomatic, but not a causal correlation between thermal tests and the pathological state [20, 21, 34]. Furthermore, Seltzer et al. have found that, in general, cold tests produce more reliable results than heat tests [4, 20, 21, 34]. White and

Cooley [35] suggest that a test providing a rapid thermal change is more desirable than a gradual temperature change. The patient is instructed to raise their hand as soon as they feel any sensation, and leave their hand up as long as the sensation lasts. The stimulus is removed and the time recorded.

Cold

Ice sticks, spray refrigerants, and carbon dioxide (CO_2) are three materials that can be used to stimulate the pulp. Cold responses appear to be related to the thickness and type of tooth structure [36]. Other factors that may affect the thermal response include a history of trauma, root development, and heavily restored teeth [37].

Ice sticks are one option. They are typically made by freezing water in used anesthetic cartridges (Fig. 13a). The main disadvantage is that the ice melts quickly and can spread to another tooth, resulting in a false response. To eliminate this problem, the tooth should be isolated and the ice placed near the cervical area rather than on the occlusal surface, where the test is most likely to give a positive response according to Peters et al. [38] (Fig. 13b). Even though the response time is relative, it should be noted to allow comparison between teeth being tested. For teeth that respond, the clinician is looking for a delayed, lingering, or extreme reaction compared to control teeth.

Refrigerants such as 1,1,1,2-tetrafluroethane (Endo-Ice or HFC 134a) (Hygenic,® EndoIce,® Coltene/Whaledent, USA) also provide an easy

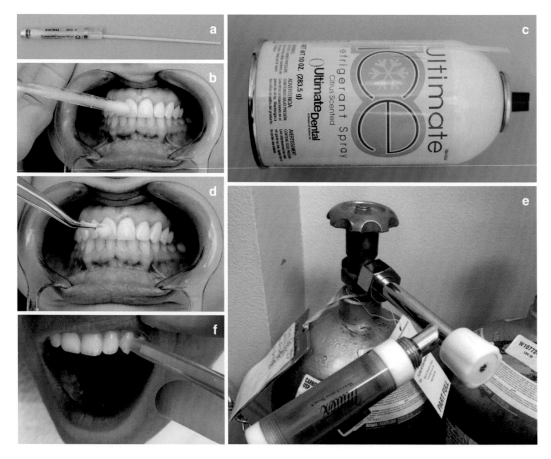

Fig. 13 Cold tests. (**a**) Ice. (**b**) Clinical use of ice. (**c**) Refrigerant. (**d**) Clinical use of refrigerant. (**e**) CO_2. (**f**) Clinical use of CO_2

manner for testing the patient's response to cold. It is colder than ice at $-26\ ^{\circ}\text{C}$ and is available in a spray canister (Fig. 13c). These refrigerants should not be sprayed directly on the tooth but should be sprayed on a cotton ball until saturated and then the cotton ball placed on the teeth being tested (Fig. 13d). Jones [39] evaluated different types of carriers for Endo-Ice and found that the greatest temperature change was recorded when a large cotton pellet was used compared to a smaller cotton pellet, a cotton tip applicator, or a cotton roll. Miller et al. [37] compared three commonly used cold tests on teeth with various restorations. The results of his work showed intact premolars and teeth restored with PFM or all-ceramic restorations responded similarly. He concluded that Endo-Ice was the most effective method for testing teeth restored with gold, PFM, and all-ceramic when the stimulus was applied for less than 15 s. If the test was longer, the Endo-Ice produced a greater decrease in temperature than CO_2. A study by Jones et al. compared response times of spray refrigerants and carbon dioxide and found that both gave equivalent pulpal responses regardless of the tooth tested or presence/absence of restorations. However, the CO_2 took significantly longer to evoke a response [40].

Carbon dioxide is also used extensively. Based on the work of Obwegeser and Steinhauser, Ehrmann [4] recommends CO_2 as the agent of choice for testing pulp vitality. The temperature typically ranges from -56 to $-98\ ^{\circ}\text{C}$ and this test is considered by many to provide the most reliable results. A cylinder of liquid CO_2 and a tube with a plunger are attached to a tank (Fig. 13e). As the liquid CO_2 passes through the orifice, is compressed with a plunger to generate an ice pencil which is then applied to the teeth (Fig. 13f). It is possible to test multiple teeth with a single cartridge and coolant placement is very well controlled. When evaluating young patients, the EPT was found to be less reliable than CO_2 and Endo-Ice. However, for adult patients, there was no statistical difference between refrigerant, CO_2, and EPT [28]. The initial cost of procuring a tank is a consideration for using this technique. Following a concern that the extreme cold might damage the enamel by causing cracks to the tooth surface, studies by Peters et al. [41] as well as Ingram and Peters [42] have shown that application of CO_2 to the tooth did not damage the tooth surface.

Heat

The application of heat to a tooth causes a slower reaction than cold due to stimulation of the unmyelinated C fibers resulting in a longer sensation. Jafarzadeh and Abbot discuss the methods of delivery and conclude that heat tests are infrequently performed because of the difficulty associated with isolation and obtaining a consistent heat source. Furthermore, they cite multiple studies which studies show the poor diagnostic accuracy of this test [7]. Heated gutta percha, heated hand instruments, electrical heat sources, frictional heat application, and heated water baths have all been used with varying results.

Gutta percha (Fig. 14a) or stopping compound (Fig. 14b) can be heated and placed on the teeth that have been prepared by drying and then lightly coated with petroleum jelly. Rickoff et al. recommend that heat should not be applied in this way for more than 5 s [43]. The difficulty in maintaining a constant known temperature of the gutta percha as well as isolation especially in the posterior region has made this test of limited value.

Hand instruments can be heated over a flame and then placed on the tooth. However, the temperature is unknown, and the risk of burning the soft tissue is substantial. Therefore, this method is not recommended. The hot water bath is another technique that allows for very little control over the temperature and the possibility of burning the patient, as it is difficult to keep the liquid from touching other tissues.

Perhaps the best option for consistent heat delivery is an electric source. A heat source is set at the manufacturer's recommendation using the appropriate delivery tip. As with the gutta percha, the tip is then placed on the tooth that has been dried and lightly lubricated. The temperature is not adjusted or increased, and 150 °F has been determined to be a safe temperature that will not result in damage to the hard or soft tissue [7].

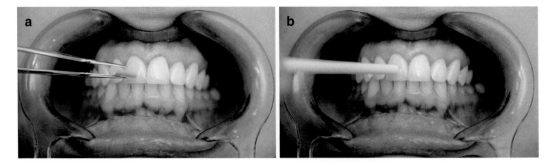

Fig. 14 Heat tests. (**a**) Gutta percha application. (**b**) Stopping compound application

Five techniques, including heated gutta percha, heated ball burnisher, hot water, and two electronic heat sources were evaluated by Bierma et al. [44]. Results suggest that hot water or a heated ball burnisher provided the most rapid response which could be useful when attempting to evoke a response from teeth that did not respond to milder stimuli. However, the heated gutta percha and electronic methods were found to be the safest in terms of preventing damage to healthy tissue. In the end, it is important that the clinician remains vigilant when applying a heat source to the dentition so as not to damage normal tissue.

Other Thermal Tests

Surface Temperature
In 1978, Banes and Hammond [9] evaluated a method to reliably assess the vitality of teeth. The premise of their study was that teeth with no vital pulp tissue would have a surface temperature that was significantly and measurably lower than vital teeth. They used a thermistor and evaluated matched pairs of vital and non-vital teeth. Their results confirmed the earlier works of Howell and others as well as Stoops and Scott [45] that non-vital teeth did indeed demonstrate a surface temperature measurably lower than vital teeth. The only exception was teeth restored with full gold coverage, where there was no difference between temperatures of vital vs. non-vital teeth. The authors concluded that restorative materials presented the greatest difficulty in measuring tooth surface temperature.

Fanibunda [46] also studied whether tooth vitality could be determined by crown surface temperature. He introduced a device consisting of two matched thermistors connected back-to-back, allowing one to measure the temperature of the crown and the other to act as a control. His results were not able to support the hypothesis that each tooth type would have a specific temperature range. However, he was able to show that after cooling the tooth surface, there was a correlation between time to rewarm and tooth vitality. Unfortunately, the time needed to acquire the measurements and the sensitivity of the technique to mouth breathing make this technique difficult to use in a clinical setting.

Some 20 years later, Smith et al. [47] re-evaluated the studies of Fanibunda regarding the validity of using tooth temperature to assess the vitality of human pulp tissue. After both in vitro and in vivo experiments, Smith concluded there were too many variables to allow meaningful clinical use of this approach.

Plethysmography
A plethysmograph is an instrument that measures changes in volume within an organ, usually resulting from fluctuation in the volume of blood that it contains. First mentioned by Reich in 1952, it has been described by several other names. The technique involves passing light through a tooth and measuring the amount of light transmitted through the tooth at specific wavelengths of light using a photocell and galvanometer. Hemoglobin selectively absorbs certain wavelengths of light such that warmth or inflammation-related vasodilation results in increased selective light absorption by

hemoglobin. While theoretically feasible, the technique's reliability has yet to be established. At the time of Pitt Ford's evaluation of available techniques for the determination of pulp status [48], he noted only one investigation that was able to demonstrate a successful application in dentistry.

Schmitt et al. [49] proposed a study to investigate the influence of tooth size, detector position, and wavelength to develop an instrument that can be used to distinguish between vital and non-vital teeth. Using a prototype device that measured diffuse light transmission at 575 nm, they were able to demonstrate that plethysmography showed promise as an objective and noninvasive diagnostic method for clinically assessing pulp vitality.

Electronic Thermography

Gratt and Sickles [50] evaluated the possibility of using electronic thermography as a diagnostic test for patients with complex diagnostic issues. Computerized electronic thermography is a rapid, noninvasive, nonionizing method of obtaining information based on heat emission from facial structures. Thermography is based on the presumption that body temperature is maintained in a homeostasis, allowing vascular changes to be detected before structural changes occur. Components include an infrared scanner, control unit, thermal image computer, software, cables, stands, supports, and color monitors with a camera and printer. The unit may require liquid nitrogen cooling. Electronic thermography has been determined to be a safe adjunctive procedure for use in the diagnosis of select neurologic and musculoskeletal conditions. At the time of this study, thermography has not shown to be useful in discriminating between common dental problems and should only be considered an investigational procedure. Continued research in this area may allow future clinicians to identify pathologic conditions which have no other explanation.

Nonionizing Optical Methods Employed for Diagnosis

Teeth that have undergone trauma may not respond to the typical tests in the clinician's arsenal [28, 32]. Trauma may result in resorption when the tooth is not treated endodontically, or if it is treated unnecessarily this will result in devitalization and subsequent arrested root development. Both these situations are more serious when the teeth involved have not reached complete development. A method that can inform on pulpal blood flow may overcome some of the inherent problems of previously described methods that attempt to determine vitality. Two techniques show great promise and several others show promise, but require further research.

Pulse Oximetry (PO)

In 1975, the pulse oximeter was introduced. Its development is credited to a Japanese bioengineer, T. Aoyagi. Pulse oximetry is a noninvasive and nonionizing technique used to measure oxygen saturation in the blood. It is based on the Beer–Lambert law, which defines the linear relationship between absorbance and concentration of an absorbing species. The pulse oximeter applies this principle to measuring hemoglobin oxygenation within the blood [51]. As perfusion is a measure of pulpal vitality, and as adequate perfusion correlates with maximum oxygenation levels, this approach provides an objective method of quantifying pulpal vitality. Gopikrishna [52] described the technology as consisting of as two light-emitting diodes, one that transmits red light (640 nm) and one that transmits infrared light (940 nm). A photodetector is placed on the opposite side of the vascular bed as the light source (Fig. 15). It is the difference in absorption of oxygenated vs. deoxygenated hemoglobin that allows the pulse oximeter to determine the oxygen saturation levels, providing a direct and measurable assessment of pulp tissue vitality. The finger probe most often used for oxygen saturation is not ideal for intra-oral testing because of the curvature of the dentition, which affects access and a linear light path. Schnettler [53] evaluated a new probe design to take this curvature into account and found pulse oximetry to be a reliable and noninvasive method to diagnose pulp vitality. Calil et al. [54] reported that the oxygen saturation level of vital pulp tissue as

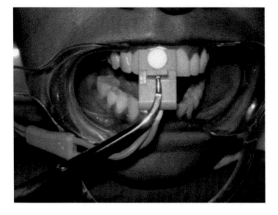

Fig. 15 Pulse oximeter dental probe placed on patient's tooth

determined using a specifically configured dental probe was consistently less than that determined using a finger probe.

Therefore the only appropriate use of a finger pulse oximeter in dentistry is for monitoring patients' overall health during sedation [55].

Another valuable application of pulse oximetry is the determination of pulpal status following traumatic injury. It is well recognized that traditional but indirect methods routinely used to evaluate pulpal health following trauma have provided inconsistent results [5, 6, 8, 19, 22]. Gopikrishna found that 94% of teeth recently traumatized showed pulp vitality when evaluated with a pulse oximeter starting at day zero, but when testing with thermal and EPT vitality testing did not return to normal for 3–6 months following the traumatic incident [52]. Thus pulse oximetry provides the clinician the ability to render treatment based on an accurate diagnosis without having to wait for confirmation.

Several variables may influence the reliability of the pulse oximeter. Jafarzadeh describes the critical elements to ensure reproducible and accurate results. First, the "sensor should conform to the size, shape, and anatomy of the tooth." Second, the probe should be held firmly against the tooth. And third, both the patient and the probe should be very still for the duration of the reading [51]. Pulse oximetry may provide a high reading if the patinet is hypoxic. The varying anatomy of different teeth presents additional challenges, and several authors have

developed methods to improve and stabilize probe placement. Noblett et al. [56] modified a rubber dam clamp to allow placement and removal of the sensors, insuring probe stability. They were then able to manipulate the oxygen saturation levels used, which allowed a variety of saturation levels to be evaluated for accuracy. Gopikrishna [52] also demonstrated the ability to obtain accurate results with a custom-designed probe and sensor holder (Fig. 15). With a modified ear probe, Goho [57] was able to determine that non-vital teeth recorded 0% oxygen saturation levels while vital teeth provided readings averaging 94% and the finger control provided readings of 98%.

Optical Coherence Tomography (OCT)

Optical coherence tomography was first introduced by Huang in 1991 [58]. OCT uses waves in the near infrared spectrum (wavelength of approximately 10^{-7} m). As a result, OCT is considered to be a noninvasive, nonionizing imaging technique. It is able to penetrate tissue with resolution levels from 0.5–15 μm and penetration depths of up to 2.0 mm depending upon the wavelength selected. OCT combines principles of ultrasound and microscopic imaging. Rather than sound waves, OCT uses near infrared light waves that reflect off the internal microstructure of tissues. An image is produced by scanning along the specimen, acquiring line images that enable either a 2D or a 3D image to be produced.

Otis et al. developed the first OCT system for dental use in 2000 [59]. It generated images of teeth, periodontal structures (including gingival tissue contour, sulcus depth, and connective tissue attachment), and restorative margins. Shemesh was able to evaluate the internal surface of root canal walls using OCT pullback scans (Fig. 16a) [60]. Results suggest that OCT can generate intracanal microscopic images without ionizing radiation. However, the cost of the catheter is expensive and may limit this modality. In a second study, Shemesh was also able to show both high specificity and sensitivity for the identification of vertical root fractures using OCT [61].

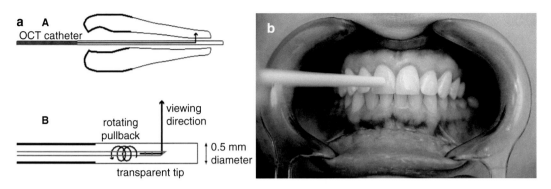

Fig. 16 OCT root canal imaging schematic. (**a**) OCT catheter inside root canal. (**b**) Rotating needle with a transparent tip situated inside catheter to serve as both a light source and receiver

A study by Braz examined the ability of OCT to identify the pulp–dentin boundary. Using a "home-built" spectral OCT system, images were obtained for comparison with histologic findings [62]. Braz et al. reported that all structural components of the pulp–dentin complex were identified in OCT and confirmed by comparison with histologic images. Braz discusses the findings of Camp's work evaluating the importance of remaining dentin thickness after tooth preparation. The smaller the remaining dentin thickness the greater the likelihood of pulpal damage. Braz suggested that OCT can be useful during tooth preparation to avoid inadvertent pulp exposure. OCT may also be used to monitor dentin bridge formation, providing information on pulp capping success.

Laser Doppler Flowmetry (LDF)

At about the same time as the emergence of OCT, laser Doppler flowmetry (LDF) was being developed to measure blood flow. First developed for medical applications, it was not long until dentists saw the value of an accurate and reproducible method to determine pulpal blood flow as a measure of pulpal vitality and as a basis for treatment planning in the patient.

LDF uses either an infrared (780–820 nm) or near infrared (632.8 nm) beam of light that is directed at the target tissue through optical fibers. The light source will hit both the stationary cells and any moving cells, and photons will scatter

these cells differently. Photons that hit stationary cells will not have their frequency shifted, while photons scattered by the moving cells will shift the frequency of absorbed light in agreement with the Doppler principle. The light containing both the shifted and non-shifted cells is backscattered to a photodetector. The outcome signal depends on the number and velocity of illuminated cells and is termed flux. Ultimately, this signal is converted based on algorithms and recorded as perfusion units (PU) (mL/min/100 g tissue). However, the perfusion unit is an arbitrary unit and varies according to the software of each instrument [63]. As a result, the PU cannot be compared between instruments or even on the same unit unless the instruments have been calibrated.

To improve the objectivity of the results of LDF, a technique known as fast Fourier transform (FFT) analysis can be applied. FFT identifies the presence of consistency of time between peaks in pulses of the LDF, confirming vitality.

In 1986, Gazelius [64] was the first to demonstrate that LDF could differentiate between vital and non-vital pulp tissue in humans. This was based on a small sample where a patient's heart rate (measured by electrocardiogram) was compared to the peak of flow measured first in healthy teeth and then again in teeth that had been injected with anesthetic containing epinephrine. The injection of epinephrine resulted in a pronounced and long-lasting reduction in values. In a later case report, Gazelius was able to show in injured teeth with no flux at the time of initial injury, after 6 weeks LDF showed an incomplete return of pulpal blood flow. Nine months after traumatic injury, the teeth showed a normal response to both LDF and electrical stimulation, with the EPT indicating a return to normal [65].

Wilder-Smith [66] in 1988, applied noninvasive laser Doppler flowmetry as a method to examine differences in pulpal blood flow (PBF) of the various types of teeth and to monitor the influence of carious lesions at 3 and 14 days post restoration. Results of her work show that PBF of teeth with minimal carious invasion did not change significantly from that of control teeth with no carious lesions, confirming the histological findings of Massler [67]. Furthermore, teeth with deep lesions demonstrated an increase in PBF which was also supported by histological findings of Brannstrom and Massler [67, 68]. These results support the correlation of deep caries and pulpal inflammation. Teeth that did not improve over 14 days, suggesting severe pulpal damage, were re-evaluated after 2 months. Five of the six teeth demonstrated minimal PBF levels, and three showed no response to electric or thermal stimuli. Based on these early findings, it seems clear that PBF can be used to assess the state of the pulp tissue and consequently can be a valuable adjunctive method to aid in pulpal diagnosis. Yanpiset [69] in 2001 was able to definitively show that LDF can correctly predict pulpal status using histological parameters. He found LDF readings correctly predicted the pulp status as vital or non-vital in 83.7% of the teeth evaluated, 73.9% for vital pulp, and 95% for those teeth that were non-vital.

One of the obstacles to reproducing consistent results over time is the difficulty in placing the probe in the same location for each test. One solution is to fabricate a custom-made stent. This will ensure that the probe is placed in the same location and orientation at each appointment. However, there are several possible shortcomings to using a custom stent. First, if the patient presents with a recent history of trauma, it may not be possible to make an impression at that appointment. Second, if there is any mobility in the dentition, the stent may not fit accu-

rately on subsequent visits. Third, if the patient is undergoing orthodontic treatment, it may be difficult to fabricate a stent because of the brackets and tooth movement. There may also be a problem with storage of the stent as well as warpage over time, depending on the material used. Differences in the actual probe design were evaluated by Ingolfsson et al. [70]. He looked at the separation and orientation of fibers within the probe and found the probe design with the largest separation between fibers was the design that produced the higher output. However, contradicting results were reported in subsequent studies by Ingolfsson [71] as well as Odor [72].

Soo-ampom et al. found that interference from other tissues such as the gingiva can generate a confounding positive output signal when testing teeth with necrotic pulp tissue [73]. To minimize this interference, it has been recommended to place a rubber dam over the teeth to be evaluated prior to fitting the customized stent.

Difficulties encountered by probe design, probe placement, and/or tissue interference are easily addressed theoretically. However, in spite of the well-documented potential of LDF in dentistry, it has not been adopted for endodontic diagnosis in clinical practice.

Ultrasound

Ultrasound technology may not be as valuable as LDF or pulse oximetry in detecting pulpal blood flow. However, if there is an apical lesion, ultrasound may be able to contribute to a more accurate diagnosis, directing potential treatment options. Because it is non-ionizing, it is considered a safe technique for evaluating soft tissues.

As its name implies, ultrasound imaging produces an image from sound rather than light. It involves the production of a sound wave, receiving the echo, and the formation and display of the resulting image. In addition, ultrasound requires a medium for transmission. Sound waves are produced by a piezoelectric transducer (the probe) at a frequency between 1 and 18 MHz. The sound is focused and produces an arc-shaped wave from the transducer face. The wave then travels into the body and focuses at the desired depth. The sound wave is reflected back to the same probe based on the tissue encountered. The sound wave that returns vibrates the transducer, and this component turns the vibrations into electrical pulses that go to a scanner, where they are processed and form a digital, real-time 3D image. The image is formed by the difference in time for the wave to return and the strength of the echo [74]. As the probe is moved, a new image is generated. Between 30 and 50 images can be obtained per second. Areas such as bone are characterized as hyperechoic because the tissue has a high-echo intensity, whereas soft tissue is considered hypoechoic since it displays a low-echo intensity. The greater the difference between the two tissues, the greater the amount of reflected energy and the higher the echo intensity. These areas will appear as bright spots. Interpretation of the gray values is based on comparison with normal tissue. The point of echo origination can be calculated based on the time to travel to the tissue and back [75, 76].

In addition, the ultrasound image can be enhanced by the use of color power Doppler (CPD) to determine perfusion in the tissue of interest. The Doppler ultrasound test uses the same sound waves, and the reflected wave is processed by a computer and creates a picture that represents blood flow within the vessel. This movement of blood causes a change in the pitch of the reflected sound wave [77].

A 2001 study by Cotti of apical lesions provided valuable foundational information for this technology. Results of this first study include: (1) alveolar bone appeared white due to its ability to reflect the waves; (2) roots appeared whiter and were distinguishable in three dimensions; (3) solid lesions present with various echo patterns, therefore, appeared as shades of gray; and (4) lesions filled with serous fluids appear dark [75]. A second follow-up study by Cotti concentrated on the ability of ultrasound combined with CPD to discriminate between a cyst and granuloma.

For this study, a cyst was defined as a transonic, well-defined cavity containing a fluid, surrounded by bone with no evidence of vascularization. A granuloma was a lesion that was either echogenic or had a mixed content, vague bony contours and the presence of vasculature [77]. Results of this study indicated near complete agreement with the matching histology, confirming that ultrasound technology was sensitive enough to distinguish between a cyst and granuloma. Gundappa compared ultrasound, digital, and conventional radiography to evaluate their ability to correctly identify the nature of periapical lesions. The digital and conventional films were unable to differentiate the nature of the lesion. Ultrasound diagnosis was in agreement with the histologic exam in all 15 cases, but underestimated the extent of the lesion [78]. Aggarwal compared the use of CT scans and ultrasound to differentiate between cysts and granulomas and found that in all 12 cases the preoperative diagnosis by CT and ultrasound coincided with the histopathological diagnosis [79].

More recently, attention has been directed to the evaluation of healing following endodontic therapy. Rajendran followed five patients for 6 months and found that ultrasound with Doppler was useful for monitoring the healing process [80]. Even though this study included a small sample size and a short follow-up period, the results demonstrated that US could be an effective tool that is nonhazardous and accurate when used to monitor the healing of lesions of endodontic origin. This was confirmed by Tikku who found ultrasound with color Doppler was significantly better than conventional radiography in detecting changes in healing. This is because radiographs are of limited value in the detection of early bone regeneration. There did not appear to be any statistically significant difference in the mean percentage change when comparing the color Doppler and ultrasonography at either 1 week or 6 months, indicating both were valuable methods of evaluating bone healing compared to conventional radiographs [81].

One of the problems encountered when using ultrasound Doppler to measure pulpal blood flow included the inability to transmit sufficient energy to detect the small Doppler frequency shift of the slow-moving pulpal blood flow, as well as the inability to penetrate hard tissue. These challenges have been partially overcome by the recent development of high-frequency ultrasonic devices. Yoon was able to demonstrate the value of ultrasound Doppler imaging to determine pulpal blood flow. Results showed a significant difference based on multiple parameters, with root-filled teeth showing a linear and non-pulsed waveform compared to vital teeth that showed a waveform that is characteristic of an arteriole. Another advantage of using ultrasound Doppler is that unlike the pulse oximeter, it does not need a special probe that has to be stabilized on the tooth [82].

Because of its non-invasive nature, ultrasound can be used repeatedly. It is also an option for patients in whom MRI is contraindicated due to cardiac pacemakers. And it can now be used for the evaluation of both hard and soft tissues. Disadvantages include difficulty in positioning the probe when evaluating posterior areas of the oral cavity. Furthermore, ultrasound has usually been applied to superficial tissues because the bone features of the face tend to shield the deeper tissues. A practical disadvantage is that the correct interpretation of ultrasound images currently requires a trained radiologist with extensive experience [83].

Magnetic Resonance Imaging (MRI)

The invention of magnetic resonance imaging was credited to Paul Lauterbur and Mansfield in 1971. This imaging technique relies on a strong magnetic field rather than radiation. Most MRI machines are graded on the strength of the magnet, which is measured in Tesla (T) units. In vivo MRI applications range between 1.5 and 3 Tesla units. MRI techniques are founded on the principle that individual atomic nuclei can absorb or emit radio frequency energy when placed in an external magnetic field. Hydrogen atoms are most frequently used because they exist naturally

in biological organisms—in particular, the soft tissues—and can generate a detectable radio frequency. When a patient is placed within the magnetic field, the hydrogen atoms will align the protons along the long axis of the magnetic field and the patient's body. The application of a radio-frequency pulse depolarizes the hydrogen atoms and the energy released is detected [74]. By manipulation of parameters that introduce variations or gradients in the magnetic field strength in a biological sample, contrasts may be generated between different tissues and converted into two- and three-dimensional images.

The superior ability of MRI to distinguish soft tissue lesions makes it ideal for the detection of odontogenic cysts and tumors [83]. Eggars found that MRI scans do not appear to be as affected by metallic restorations when compared to CT images [84]. Idiyatullin was able to evaluate a new MRI technique, Sweep Imaging with Fourier Transform (SWIFT) to visualize dental tissue. The SWIFT images were compared with conventional radiographs, CBCT images, gradient-echo MRI, and histologic sections. It was found that SWIFT images had the potential to image minute dental structures within clinically relevant scan times, offering the endodontist a promising method to longitudinally evaluate teeth that have undergone regenerative procedures [85].

Current disadvantages of MRI involve long scanning times, high hardware cost and limited access to radiology units. While MRI appears to be a safe imaging technique, the high cost of the procedure currently makes its value limited to cases where its use is essential for a correct diagnosis.

Summary

A summary of the most frequently used diagnostic tests and those on the horizon is provided in Table 3. It is intended as a guide to assist the clinician in developing a diagnosis and treatment plan for every patient, understanding that patients often present with a complex variety of signs and symptoms.

Table 3 Overview of testing

Test	Technique	Advantages	Disadvantages	Comment
Periapical disease				
Palpation	Use finger or cotton tip applicator; apply increasing pressure in area of tooth apex	Little to no equipment needed. Easy to perform	Test may not be conclusive for pain of endodontic origin. Results are subjective and may vary between teeth and patients	Detects soft tissue swelling or bony expansion when compared to control teeth
Percussion	Use finger or instrument, tap on tooth in question from buccal, lingual, or incisal as needed	Easy to perform. Provides good information regarding inflammation of the PDL	Difficult to consistently reproduce the amount of pressure used	Result may represent a restoration that is high in occlusion, or a coronal fracture
Pulpal sensibility				
Electronic pulp testing	Isolate tooth in question and apply probe with conducting medium, increasing current until patient responds	Inexpensive. Easy to perform and interpret results. Good for teeth with increased amount of secondary dentin	Awkward to use in crowded dentition or in patients undergoing orthodontic treatment. Unreliable results in recently traumatized teeth or teeth with open apices	Lack of response is suggestive of a necrotic pulp. Concern regarding patients with cardiac pacemakers
Cold	Using instrument of choice, isolate tooth and apply cold to tooth until patient gives either a positive response or indicates no sensation to cold	More reliable in young teeth than EPT. CO_2 seems to provide most reliable result	Response time is relative. Response is subjective. Initial cost of CO_2 system. Concern of microfracture with extreme cold	Difficult to gain dependable results with heavily restored teeth. Response to cold generally has a diagnosis of irreversible pulpitis, nonresponsive teeth frequently suffer from irreversible pulpitis or pulpal necrosis
Heat	With tooth isolated, apply heat source until patient responds		Poor diagnostic accuracy. Difficulty maintaining constant temperature	
Surface temperature	Place two thermistors on tooth and record difference upon cooling	Ability to show a correlation of time to rewarm the tooth and vitality	Time needed to acquire measurements and sensitivity make technique difficult to use clinically	Full coverage restorations may affect results
Plethysmography	Using a probe, light is passed through the tooth at different wavelengths	Apparatus measures changes in blood volume	Reliability of technique has not been established clinically	
Pulpal vitality				
Pulse oximetry	A probe with two diodes is placed on the tooth to measure oxygenated and deoxygenated hemoglobin	Useful in determination of pulpal status following traumatic injury	Technique sensitive	The curvature of the tooth and dental arch results in a false reading because of the distortion of the beam as it passes through a convex surface.

(continued)

Table 3 (continued)

Test	Technique	Advantages	Disadvantages	Comment
Laser Doppler flowmetry	Apply probe to tooth surface as far removed from gingival tissue as possible	Immediate and real-time read out of data	Picks up signal from periodontal blood flow. Extremely technique sensitive. Measurements are not reproducible	Challenging for use in clinical setting
Ultrasound	Place probe with transmission medium on tooth surface to initiate sound wave	Ease of use	Low resolution, poor image quality	Limited hard tissue penetration
Magnetic resonance imaging	Patient is placed within a magnetic field where hydrogen atoms will align the protons along the long axis of the magnetic field and patient's body	Superior ability to distinguish soft tissue lesions such as cysts and tumors	Procedure most often performed at an imaging center. Expensive	Scans not as affected by metal when compared to CT images
Test cavity	With no anesthesia, a small class I cavity is prepared	If patient reports a sensation, presumption of vitality	Irreversible procedure. Increased patient anxiety	Unlikely to provide definitive information, especially in case of extreme calcification or heavily restored tooth
Selective anesthesia	Using a small amount of anesthetic, inject near target site	Useful as a tool to rule out pain of endodontic origin	Can only be used when the patient presents with pain at the time of examination	May be useful in determining pain of non-odontogenic origin such as cardiac, TMD, referred or neural origin
Miscellaneous				
Transillumination	Apply light source to buccal and lingual surface	Easy to perform and accurate	Rarely useful when testing a tooth that has been heavily restored	Most useful in the identification of cusp or marginal ridge fracture. Extent of fracture may be difficult to determine
Bite	Instruct patient to bite firmly then release quickly from instrument	Easy and convenient for both patient and clinician to use	Result may be subjective	Provides anatomical specific response
Optical coherence	Apply imaging probe to the tooth or inside root canal	Real-time high-resolution imaging	Imaging depth may be inadequate to view the entire dental pulp structure. Cost may be a limiting factor	

Conclusion

Endodontic therapy is performed for a variety of reasons. Foremost is the alleviation of pain and pathosis. However, a patient may experience trauma necessitating endodontic therapy, or a complex restorative plan may call for intentional endodontic therapy. In any case, prior to initiating treatment, an accurate diagnosis must be determined. A thorough understanding of the biology of the pulp is needed as well. The testing modalities currently available to the clinician will provide information necessary to develop an accurate diagnosis. In addition, the patient must be informed of the anticipated prognosis, which may include alternative treatment modalities, such as extraction and restoration of function with an implant, bridge, or removable partial denture.

Unfortunately, the most frequently used diagnostic tests only give the practitioner a suggestion of the actual status of tooth health and vitality. With current advances in science and technology, more precise techniques will make their way into endodontic and general dental practices, enabling more accurate diagnoses, better endodontic outcomes and overall improved oral health.

References

1. Robinson HGB. The nature of the diagnostic process. Dent Clin North Am. 1963;3:3–8.
2. Berman LH, Rotstein I. Diagnosis. In: Hargreaves KM, Berman LH, editors. Cohen's pathways of the pulp. 11th ed. Maryland Heights: Mosby; 2016. p. 5.
3. Chambers IG. The role and methods of pulp testing in oral diagnosis: a review. Int Endod J. 1982;15:1–5.
4. Ehrmann EH. Pulp testers and pulp testing with particular reference to the use of dry ice. Aust Dent J. 1977;22:272–9.
5. Mumford JM, Bjorn H. Problems in electric pulp testing and dental algesimetry. Int Dent J. 1962;12:161–79.
6. Alghaithy RA, Qualtrough AJE. Pulp sensibility and vitality tests for diagnosing pulpal health in permanent teeth: a critical review. Int Endod J. 2017;50:135–72.
7. Jafarzedeh H, Abbott PV. Review of pulp sensibility tests. Part I: electric pulp tests and test cavities. Int Endod J. 2010;43:738–62.
8. Jafarzedeh H, Abbott PV. Review of pulp sensibility tests. Part II: electric pulp tests and test cavities. Int Endod J. 2010;43:945–58.
9. Banes JD, Hammond HL. Surface temperature of vital and nonvital teeth in humans. J Endod. 1978;4(4):106–9.
10. Glossary of endodontic terms. 9th ed. www.aae.org.
11. Berman LH, Rotstein I. Diagnosis. In: Hargreaves KM, Berman LH, editors. Cohen's Pathways of the Pulp. 11th ed. Maryland Heights: Mosby; 2016. p. 15.
12. O'Leary TJ. Tooth mobility. Dent Clin North Am. 1969;13(3):567–79.
13. Kulilid JC. Diagnosis of endodontic disease: B. Diagnostic testing. In: Ingle JI, Backland LK, Baumgartner JC, editors. Ingle's endodontics. 6th ed. Ontario: BC Decker; 2008. p. 539.
14. Weisman MI. The use of a calibrated percussion instrument in pulpal and periapical diagnosis. Oral Surg Oral Med Oral Pathol. 1984;57(3):320–2.
15. Hill CM. The efficacy of transillumination in vitality tests. Int Endod J. 1986;19(4):198–201.
16. Friedman J, Marcus MI. Transillumination of the oral cavity with use of fiber optics. J Am Dent Assoc. 1970;80(4):801–9.
17. Berman LH, Rotstein I. Diagnosis. In: Hargreaves KM, Berman LH, editors. Cohen's pathways of the pulp. 11th ed. Maryland Heights: Mosby; 2016. p. 20.
18. Kulilid JC. Diagnosis of endodontic disease: B. Diagnostic testing. In: Ingle JI, Backland LK, Baumgartner JC, editors. Ingle's endodontics. 6th ed. Ontario: BC Decker; 2008. p. 542.
19. Nahri MV, Virtanen A, Kuhta J, Huopaniemi T. Electrical stimulation of teeth with a pulp tester in the cat. Scand J Dent Res. 1979;87:32–8.
20. Seltzer S, Bender IB, Ziontz M. The dynamics of pulp inflammation: correlations between diagnostic data and actual histologic findings in the pulp. Part I. Oral Surg Oral Med Oral Pathol. 1963;16:846–71.
21. Seltzer S, Bender IB, Ziontz M. The dynamics of pulp inflammation: correlations between diagnostic data and actual histologic findings in the pulp. Part II. Oral Surg Oral Med Oral Pathol. 1963;16: 969–77.
22. Peterson K, Soderstrom C, Kiani-Anaraki M, Levy G. Evaluation of the ability of thermal and electric tests to register pulp vitality. Endod Dent Traumatol. 1999;15:127.
23. Myers JW. Demonstration of a possible source of error with an electric pulp tester. J Endod. 1998;24:199–200.
24. Anderson RW, Pantera EA. Influence of a barrier technique on electric pulp testing. J Endod. 1988;14(4):179–80.
25. Michaelson RE, Seidberg BH, Guttuso J. An in vivo evaluation of interface media used with the electric pulp tester. J Am Dent Assoc. 1975;91(1):118–21.
26. Bender IB, Landau MA, Fonsecca S, Trowbridge HO. The optimum placement site of the electrode in electric pulp testing of the 12 anterior teeth. J Am Dent Assoc. 1989;118(3):305–10.
27. Jacobson JJ. Probe placement during electric pulp testing procedures. Oral Surg Oral Med Oral Pathol. 1984;58(2):242–7.
28. Fuss Z, Trowbridge H, Bender IB, Rickoff B, Sorin S. Assessment of reliability of electrical and thermal pulp testing agents. J Endod. 1986;12(7):301–5.
29. Woolley LH, Woodworth J, Dobbs JL. A preliminary evaluation of the effects of electrical pulp testers on dogs with artificial pacemakers. J Am Dent Assoc. 1974;89(5):1099–101.
30. Wilson BL, Broberg C, Baumgartner JC, et al. Safety of electronic apex locators and pulp testers in patients with implanted cardiac pacemakers or cardioverter/ defibrillators. J Endod. 2006;32(9):847–52.

31. Simon AB, Linde B, Bonnette GH, Schlentz RJ. The individual with a pacemaker in the dental environment. J Am Dent Assoc. 1975;91(6):1224–9.

32. Fulling HJ, Andreasen JO. Influence of maturation status and tooth type of permanent teeth upon electrometric and thermal pulp testing. Scand J Dent Res. 1976;84(5):286–90.

33. Hyman JJ, Cohen ME. The predictive value of endodontic diagnostic tests. Oral Surg Oral Med Oral Pathol. 1984;58:343–6.

34. Reynolds RL. The determination of pulp vitality by means of thermal and electrical stimuli. Oral Surg Oral Med Oral Pathol. 1966;22(2):231–40.

35. White JH, Cooley RL. A quantitative evaluation of thermal pulp testing. J Endod. 1977;3(12):453–7.

36. Kulilid JC. Diagnosis of endodontic disease: B. Diagnostic testing. In: Ingle JI, Backland LK, Baumgartner JC, editors. Ingle's endodontics. 6th ed. Ontario: BC Decker; 2008. p. 534.

37. Miller SO, Johnson JD, Allemang JD, Strother JM. Cold testing through full coverage restorations. J Endod. 2004;30(10):695–700.

38. Peters DD, Baumgartner JC, Lorton L. Adult pulpal diagnosis I. Evaluation of the positive and negative responses to cold and electrical pulp tests. J Endod. 1994;20(10):506–11.

39. Jones DM. Effect of the type carrier used on the results of dichlorodifluromethane application to teeth. J Endod. 1999;25(10):692–4.

40. Jones VR, Rivera EM, Walton RE. Comparison of CO2 versus refrigerant spray to determine pulpal responsiveness. J Endod. 2002;28(7):531–3.

41. Peters DD, Mader CL, Donnelly JC. Evaluation of the effects of carbon dioxide used as a pulpal test 3. In vivo effect on human enamel. J Endod. 1986;12(1):13–20.

42. Ingram TA, Peters DD. Evaluation of the effects of carbon dioxide used as a pulpal test. 2. In vivo effect on canine enamel and pulpal tissues. J Endod. 1983;9(7):296–303.

43. Rickoff B, Trowbridge H, Baker J, Fuss Z, Bender IB. Effects of thermal vitality tests on human dental pulp. J Endod. 1988;14:482–5.

44. Bierma MM, McClanaham S, Baisden MK, Bowles WR. Comparison of heat-testing methodology. J Endod. 2012;38(8):1106–9.

45. Stoops LC, Scott D. Measurement of tooth temperature as a means of determining pulp vitality. J Endod. 1976;2(5):141–5.

46. Fanibunda KB. The feasibility of temperature measurement as a diagnostic procedure in human teeth. J Dent. 1986;14:126–9.

47. Smith E, Dickson M, Evans AL, Smith D, Murray CA. An evaluation of the use of tooth temperature to assess human pulp vitality. Int Endod J. 2004;37:374–80.

48. Pitt Ford TR, Patel S. Technical equipment for assessment of dental pulp status. Endod Topics. 2004;7:2–13.

49. Schmitt JM, Walker EC, Webber RL. Optical determination of dental pulp vitality. IEEE Trans Biomed Eng. 1991;38(4):346–52.

50. Gratt BM, Sickles EA. Future applications of electronic thermography. J Am Dent Assoc. 1991;122(5):28–36.

51. Jafarzadeh H, Rosenberg PA. Pulse oximetry: review of a potential aid in endodontic diagnosis. J Endod. 2009;35(3):329–33.

52. Gopikrishna V, Tinagupta K, Kandaswamy D. Comparison of electrical, thermal, and pulse oximetry methods for assessing pulp vitality in recently traumatized teeth. J Endod. 2007;33:531–5.

53. Schnettler JM, Wallace JA. Pulse oximetry as a diagnostic tool of pulpal vitality. J Endod. 1991;17(10):488–90.

54. Calil E, Calderia CI, Gavini G, Lemos EM. Determination of pulp vitality in vivo with pulse oximetry. Int Endod J. 2008;41:741–73.

55. Gandy SR. The use of pulse oximetry in dentistry. J Am Dent Assoc. 1995;126:1274–8.

56. Noblett WC, Wilcox LR, Scamman F, et al. Detection of pulpal circulation in vitro by pulse oximetry. J Endod. 1995;22:1–5.

57. Goho C. Pulse oximetry evaluation of vitality in primary and immature permanent teeth. Pediatr Dent. 1999;21:125–7.

58. Huang D, Swanson EA, Lin CP, et al. Optical coherence tomography. Science. 1991;254:1178–81.

59. Otis L, Everett MJ, Sathyam US, Colston BW Jr. Optical coherence tomography: a new imaging technology for dentistry. J Am Dent Assoc. 2000;131(4):511–4.

60. Shemesh H, van Soest G, Wu MK, van der Sluis LWM, Wesselink PR. The ability of optical coherence tomography to characterize the root canal walls. J Endod. 2007;33:1369–73.

61. Shemesh H, van Soest G, Wu MK, Wesselink PR. Diagnosis of vertical root fractures with optical coherence tomography. J Endod. 2008;34:739–42.

62. Braz AK, Kyotoku BB, Gomes AS. In vitro tomographic image of human pulp-dentin complex: optical coherence tomography and histology. J Endod. 2009;35(9):1218–21.

63. Sigurdsson A. Diagnosis of endodontic disease: C. Laser Doppler flowmetry. In: Ingle JI, Backland LK, Baumgartner JC, editors. Ingle's endodontics. 6th ed. Ontario: BC Decker; 2008. p. 547–53.

64. Gazelius B, Olgart L, Edwall B, Edwall L. Noninvasive recording of blood flow in human dental pulp. Endod Dent Traumatol. 1986;2:19–21.

65. Gazelius B, Olgart L, Edwall B. Recorded vitality in luxated teeth assessed by laser Doppler flowmeter. Endod Dent Traumatol. 1988;4:265–8.

66. Wilder-Smith PFFB. A new method for the noninvasive measurement of pulpal blood flow. Int Endod J. 1988;21:307–12.

67. Massler M. Pulpal reactions to dental caries. Int Dent J. 1967;17:441–60.

68. Brannstrom M. Dentinal and pulpal response II. Application of an air stream to exposed dentine. Short observation period. An experimental study. Acta Odontol Scand. 1960;18:17–28.

69. Yanpiset K, Vangsavan N, Sigurdsson A, Trope M. Efficacy of laser Doppler flowmetry for the diagnosis of revascularization of reimplanted immature don teeth. Dental Traumatol. 2001;17:63–70.

70. Ingolfsson AR, Tronstad L, Hersh EV, Riva CE. Effect of probe design on the suitability of laser Doppler flowmetry in vitality testing of human teeth. Endod Dent Traumatol. 1993;9:65–70.

71. Ingolfsson AR, Tronstad L, Hersh EV, Riva CE. Efficacy of laser Doppler flowmetry in determining pulp vitality of human teeth. Endod Dent Traumatol. 1994;10:83–7.

72. Odor TM, Ford TR, McDonald F. Effect of probe design and bandwidth on laser Doppler readings from vital and root-filled teeth. Med Eng Phys. 1996;18:359–64.

73. Soo-ampon S, Vongsavan N, Soo-ampon M, et al. The source of laser Doppler blood flow signals recorded from human teeth. Arch Oral Biol. 2003;48:353–60.

74. Patel S, Dawood A, Whaites E, Pitt Ford T. New dimensions in endodontic imaging: Part 1. Conventional and alternative radiographic systems. Int Endod J. 2009;42:447–62.

75. Cotti E, Campisi G, Garau V, Puddu G. A new technique for the study of periapical bone lesions: ultrasound real time imaging. Int Endod J. 2002;35:148–52.

76. Cotti E. Diagnositc imaging C. Ultrasonic imaging. In: Ingle JI, Backland LK, Baumgartner JC, editors. Ingle's endodontics. 6th ed. Ontario: BC Decker; 2008. p. 547–53.

77. Cotti E, Campisi G, Ambu R, Dettori C. Ultrasound real time imaging in the differential diagnosis of periapical lesions. Int Endod J. 2003;36:556–64.

78. Gundappa M, Ng SY, Whaites EJ. Comparison of ultrasound, digital and conventional radiography in differentiating periapical lesions. Dentomaxillofac Radiol. 2006;35:326–33.

79. Aggarwal V, Logani A, Shah N. The evaluation of computed tomography scans and ultrasounds in the differential diagnosis of periapical lesions. J Endod. 2008;34(11):1312–5.

80. Rajendran N, Sundaresan B. Efficacy of ultrasound and color power Doppler as a monitoring tooth in the healing of endodontic periapical lesions. J Endod. 2007;33:181–6.

81. Tikku AP, Kumar S, Loomba K, Chandra A, Verma P, Aggarwal R. Use of ultrasound, color Doppler imaging and radiography to monitor periapical healing after endodontic surgery. J Oral Sci. 2010;52:411–6.

82. Yoon MJ, Kim E, Lee SJ, Bae YM, Kim S, Park SH. Pulpal blood flow measurement with ultrasound Doppler imaging. J Endod. 2010;36(3):419–22.

83. Shah N, Bansal N, Logani A. Recent advances in imaging technologies in dentistry. World J Radiol. 2014;6(10):794–807.

84. Eggars G, Ricker M, Kress J, Fiebach J, Dickhaus H, Hassfeld S. Artefacts in magnetic resonance imaging caused by dental material. Magnet Resonance Materials in Physics, Biology and Medicine. 2005;18:103–11.

85. Idiyatullin D, Corum C, Moeller S, Prasad HS, Garwood M, Nixdorf DR. Dental magnetic resonance imaging: making the invisible visible. J Endod. 2011;35:1645–157.

Periodontics

Carmen Todea and Silvana Canjau

Abstract

For decades, there has been an ongoing search for clinically acceptable methods for the accurate, noninvasive diagnosis, and prognosis of periodontitis. There are several well-known inherent drawbacks with current clinical procedures. The purpose of this chapter is to summarize some of the newly emerging diagnostic approaches, namely, laser Doppler (LD) imaging, optical coherence tomography (OCT), infrared spectroscopy, and ultrasound. The history and attractive features of these new approaches are briefly illustrated, and the interesting and significant inventions related to dental applications are discussed. The particularly attractive aspects for the dental community are that some of these methods are entirely noninvasive, do not impose any discomfort to the patients during the procedure, and require no tissue to be extracted. Morphologically, some other noninvasive imaging modalities, such as OCT and ultrasound, could be employed to accurately measure probing depths and assess the status of periodontal attachment, the front-line of disease progression. These methods could either replace traditional clinical examinations for the diagnosis of periodontitis or at least serve as attractive complementary diagnostic tools. However, the potential of these techniques requires careful, informed examination given the multifactorial character of periodontal disease. Alternative modalities like microbiologic and genetic approaches are also being developed.

Flow Chart Overview of Existing Techniques, Currently Available New Minimally Invasive Imaging Methods, and View to the Future

Periodontal diseases are prevalent human diseases defined by the signs and symptoms of gingival inflammation and/or periodontal tissue destruction [1].

Periodontal disease is diagnosed after the analysis of information collected in a periodontal examination. This includes the patient's medical and dental histories, and data on the presence or absence of clinical signs of inflammation, and other signs or symptoms, including pain, ulceration, amount of observable plaque and calculus, probing depths and the extent and pattern of clinical attachment and bone loss [2].

Periodontitis is a highly prevalent chronic inflammatory disorder with a negative impact on the quality of life affecting 30–40% of the population over 35 years of age [3]. It involves the

C. Todea
University of Medicine and Pharmacy,
Timisoara, Romania

S. Canjau (✉)
Coesfeld, Germany

© Springer Nature Switzerland AG 2020

P. Wilder-Smith, J. Ajdaharian (eds.), *Oral Diagnosis*, https://doi.org/10.1007/978-3-030-19250-1_3

breakdown of tooth-supporting tissues and subsequent tooth loss and is considered a major factor in the global burden of oral diseases [4]. It has been estimated that in developed countries, approximately 50% of the adult population has gingivitis in three or four teeth at any given time and 30% has periodontitis (presence of three or more teeth with pockets of ≥4 mm) [5].

The main cause of gingival inflammation is an ecological imbalance between the oral microbial biofilm and an impaired host inflammatory response [6]. Periodontal inflammation can lead to superficial ulcers in the gingival sulcus, where blood capillaries are exposed to microbial biofilms [7]. Periodontal pathogens are trans-located and released from the sulcus into the bloodstream leading to breakdown of microcirculatory function. On the other hand, dysfunction of microcirculation may impair tissue perfusion and result in organ dysfunction [8]. Inflammatory mediators

that increase vascular permeability in microvessels with adherens junctions exert this effect by disrupting junctional complex assembly via phosphorylation, internalization, and/or degradation of junctional molecules [9]. Gingival inflammation results in an increased number of capillary loops, enlargement of the vessel size and slowing of blood flow, and limitation of the afferent blood vessels. Research indicated an interaction between gingival blood flow and gingival health [10]. Inflammatory changes of the vascular morphology are associated with blood flow changes, which may serve as early indicators of the onset of pathological events in the gingival tissues [11].

For decades, there has been an ongoing search for clinically acceptable methods for the accurate, noninvasive diagnosis, and prognosis of periodontitis. There are several well-known inherent drawbacks with current clinical procedures. The purpose of this chapter is to summa-

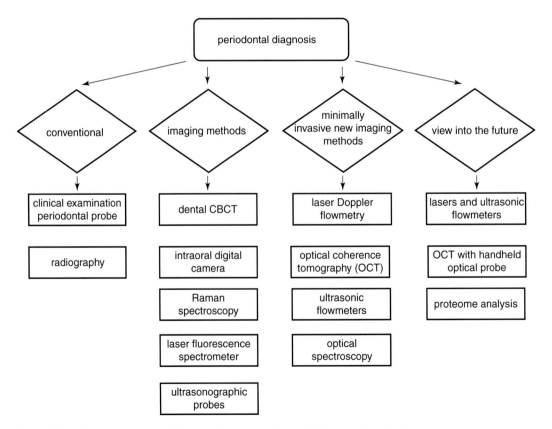

Fig. 1 Flow chart overview of existing techniques, currently available new minimally invasive imaging methods, and view to the future

rize some of the newly emerging diagnostic approaches, namely, laser Doppler (LD) imaging, optical coherence tomography (OCT), infrared spectroscopy, and ultrasound. The history and attractive features of these new approaches are briefly illustrated, and the interesting and significant inventions related to dental applications are discussed. The particularly attractive aspects for the dental community are that some of these methods are entirely noninvasive, do not impose any discomfort on the patients during the procedure, and require no tissue to be extracted. For instance, multiple inflammatory indices withdrawn from near-infrared spectra have the potential to identify early signs of inflammation leading to tissue breakdown. Morphologically, some other nonin-

vasive imaging modalities, such as OCT and ultrasound, could be employed to accurately measure probing depths and assess the status of periodontal attachment, the front-line of disease progression. Given that these methods reflect a completely different assessment of periodontal inflammation, if clinically validated, these methods could either replace traditional clinical examinations for the diagnosis of periodontitis or at least serve as attractive complementary diagnostic tools. However, the potential of these techniques requires careful, informed examination given the multifactorial character of periodontal disease. In addition to these imaging tools (Fig. 1), alternative modalities like microbiologic and genetic approaches are also being developed.

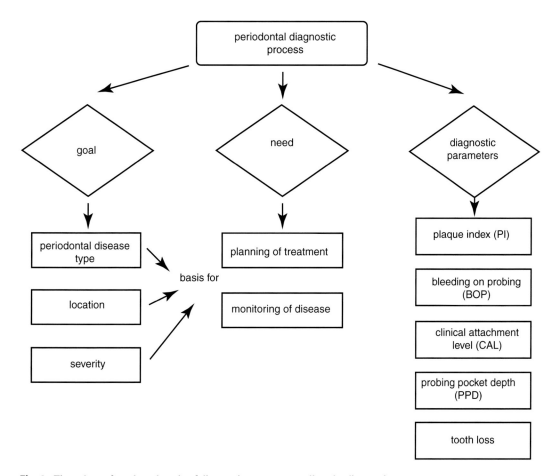

Fig. 2 Flow chart of needs and goals of diagnostic process as well as the diagnostic parameters

Need and Goal of Diagnostic Process

The goal of periodontal diagnostic procedures is to provide information to the clinician on periodontal disease type, location, and severity; this information can serve as a basis for treatment planing and monitoring [12]. Traditional diagnostic procedures are often insufficient for identifying sites of active disease, for arriving at a diagnosis and planing treatment, for quantitatively monitoring a patient's response to therapy and for measuring the degree of susceptibility to future disease progression [13] (Fig. 2). Thus, identifying susceptible individuals or sites at risk for disease and diagnosing active phases of periodontal disease are challenging for both clinicians and oral health researchers [14].

There has been increasing focus on developing more sensitive and specific diagnostic tests for periodontal diseases as a means of improving therapy [15]. Innovations such as biosensors, nanotechnology, ultrasonography, optical imaging systems, and proteome analysis of oral fluids are all being considered as potential tools for determining the health and/or disease status of patients. Several novel methods that are currently being explored as complementary tools in periodontal diagnostics are discussed in this chapter.

Principles and Devices of Minimally Invasive New Imagining Methods

Laser Doppler

Microcirculation of the Gingiva Assessed by Laser Doppler Flowmetry

There is little information in the literature about the vascular dynamics of the gingival circulation in healthy and diseased sites. Laser Doppler flowmetry (LDF) emerged more than 30 years ago as a noninvasive and real-time method for perfusion measurements [16]. LD techniques were able to demonstrate the differing blood flow wave patterns between gingival tissue types [17] and the consistency of same-subject measurements over time [18]. One of the earliest signs of

any inflammatory process is the change in vascular architecture and microvasculature. This is also true for gingivitis [19]. The healthy gingiva is characterized by a sub-epithelial vascular plexus consisting of a capillary network with loops arching towards the epithelium [20]. Gingival inflammation presents an increased vascularity with larger vessel size, more capillary loops [21], slowed blood flow [22], and a restriction of the afferent blood vessels [23]. The capillary units are among the first vessels affected by inflammation in the crestal gingiva [24]. If changes of the vascular morphology in inflammation are related to blood flow changes, they may serve as an early predictor for the onset of gingival pathology [25]. Gingival microcirculation (GM) has lacked exact evaluation for a long time. This was mainly due to methodological difficulties. Different methods, such as impedance plethysmography or the implantation of microspheres, have been employed to study GBF [26–28]. Unfortunately, most of them were invasive or inapplicable to humans. Other studies on dogs have shown that predictable morphologic changes occur in the blood vessels at the gingival margin with the onset of inflammation. These vascular changes precede recognizable histopathological alterations, starting as early as 2 days after the induction of gingivitis [29, 30]. In our studies, in order to obtain a correct LDF measurement of the gingival blood flow, the probe was positioned 4 mm above the cervical line of the upper incisors and was also distanced using a gingival dam. This distance was necessary in order to avoid pressure on the gingival tissue. A silicone rubber holder was used to secure the gingival LDF probe in position. A small hole for the laser probe was placed in the holder at 4 mm away from the gingival margin, using a high-speed handpiece and a 1.5 mm diameter fissure bur. After calibration and disinfection, the laser probe was inserted into a rigid opaque plastic tube with a 1.5 mm diameter and 0.1–0.2 mm longer than the fiber. The plastic tube was used to reduce the movement artifacts of the fiber inside the impression, by increasing adherence and protection of the active optic surface. The plastic tube was forcefully inserted in the canal carved in the impression and positioned afterwards according to study protocol. With the purpose of ensuring the reproducibility of LD signal acquisition, a guiding mark was set on the fiber in order to allow its placement in the same position for each testing.

Healthy and Inflamed Gingiva

LDF provides data on the blood flow of the marginal gingiva. However, there exists a difference in blood supply of marginal gingiva of the upper and lower jaws [31] and between blood flow at the premolars vs. molars vs. the anterior teeth. A statistically significant difference was also demonstrated between blood supply in the maxillary and the mandibular anterior gingiva in the interdental gingiva, attached gingiva, and alveolar mucosa [32]. The difference was significant for the mandibular anterior gingiva only in the alveolar mucosa region [33]. Scattering by surrounding tissues as well as morphological characteristics such as gingival thickness, in particular, periodontal biotypes, might influence LDF variability [11]. Age as well as the epithelial thickness also affect the gingival vasculature, decreasing LDF readings [34]. Mechanical stimulation of the gingiva, for example, during tooth brushing, significantly increases gingival blood flow in the papillary gingiva of healthy individuals [35].

Marginal blood flow can also be affected by restorations or plaque accumulation [36]. Vag and Fazekas investigated the effects of the crown margin on gingival health and found a correlation between gingival index and LDF results [37]. Al-Wahadni et al. found higher gingivitis levels associated with plaque accumulation on resinbonded bridges [38]. Sub-gingival restoration margins might bring forth an additional inflammatory effect on the gingival tissue resulting in higher blood flow values of test sites [9]. Nevertheless, LDF was found to have only limited diagnostic value in relation to the clinical performance of fixed prostheses [10].

The gingival microcirculation exhibits a dramatic, dynamic change in response to the development and progression of gingivitis. However, the relationship between plaque accumulation, gingival inflammation, and tissue microcirculation remains controversial. Increased blood flow in inflamed gingiva vs. healthy gingiva was demonstrated in several animal [28, 39, 40] and clinical studies [17, 32, 41, 42]. According to Kerdvongbundit et al., inflammation alters the microcirculatory and micro-morphologic dynamics of the human gingiva before and after conventional treatment (scaling and root planing); however, blood flow returned to normal after treatment and remained stable for 3-month post-treatment. However, Matheny et al. reported reduced blood flow in inflamed gingiva and an increased number of superficial vessels [43]. Other clinical studies found a positive correlation between LDF measurements and gingival inflammation or bleeding on probing [37, 44, 45].

LDF is an objective noninvasive method of monitoring the response to periodontal therapy. It can be used to quantify gingival blood flow following periodontal surgery, mapping out changing patterns of microvascular blood flow during the wound healing period [46]. The gingival blood flow decreases immediately following anesthesia and remains diminished immediately following surgery. A comparison of the gingival blood flow responses following simplified papilla preservation techniques vs. the modified Widman flap technique indicated that the first method may be associated with faster postoperative recovery of the gingival blood flow [47].

LDF techniques have been used to demonstrate the effects of smoking on gingival blood flow. In young people, a significant, immediate increase in gingival blood flow was observed during smoking that returned to baseline within 10 min [48]. It is speculated that small repeated vasoconstrictive attacks due to cigarette smoking may contribute to gingival vascular dysfunction and periodontal disease in the long run [49]. However, work by Palmer et al. does not seem to support the theory that tobacco smoking causes localized vasoconstriction in the periodontal tissues [50]. This may be due to elevation in blood pressure induced by smoking, which overcomes any vasoconstrictive effects of smoking. Mullally proposed that LDF in periodontics is only applicable in the measurement of acute changes in blood flow [51]. However, it was shown that smoking causes an acute increase in relative blood flow in the forehead skin in light smokers compared to heavy smokers, suggesting a potential induction of tolerance in regular users of tobacco [52]. Moreover, gingival blood vessels in smokers with healthy gingival conditions respond differently to administration of an anesthetic containing a vasoconstrictor in comparison with those of non-smokers [53].

Changes in gingival blood flow after orthodontic force application were also studied by the LDF technique. It was estimated that this change correlated to the degree of force applied to displace the teeth although individual responses to the same degree of force varied in dependence on the degree of tooth displacement [54] and the size of the interdental space [55]. The regression coefficient of decreased blood flow to the percentage of tooth displacement was significantly higher in young subjects than in adults. Barta et al. showed that the application of a force of 75 g to the maxillary canine in an ectopic position resulted in a decrease in gingival blood flow up to 50%, but it returned towards the baseline after a few months [56].

One of our studies [57] aimed at evaluating the microcirculation in subjects with gingivitis compared to healthy gingiva by using LDF. The subjects of the present study were young adults in whom oral hygiene and dietary habits were well established. Ramsay et al. [58] indicated that the reliability of blood flow measurements required accurate repositioning of the measurement probe; that is why the technique used in the study went to great lengths to ensure reproducibility of the LDF measurements. The results showed that

LDF could be a useful noninvasive, sensitive, reproducible, and harmless method for measuring GM in humans. LDF may therefore be an important element in clarifying the role of GBF dynamics in clinical gingivitis as well as in understanding the blood flow dynamics in the gingiva. In our study, on the the seventh day, the gingiva was not restored to a healthy condition, with normal blood flow as shown by LDF, but after 14 days, the GM recorded by LDF and the clinical assessment also showed almost a complete restoration of the gingivitis group. Consequently, the clinical signs of inflammation correlated with the changes in GBF (Fig. 3).

The results showed significant statistical differences between the four measurement time points. At 24 h after the initiation of therapy, the GBF was significantly increased compared to the baseline values, suggesting local inflammation of the tissues after the initial therapy. No significant differences were observed between the initial moment and 7 days after the treatment and also between initial moment and 14 days after. The GBF values at 14 days were not significantly different compared to the control group (Fig. 4).

Root Planing

A laser Doppler periodontal probe has recently been developed for intrasulcular measurement of gingival blood flow. The specific aims of one investigation [45] were to determine the relation between intrasulcular laser Doppler readings

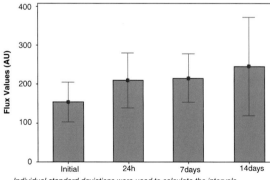
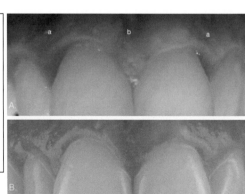

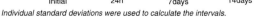

Individual standard deviations were used to calculate the intervals.

Fig. 3 The mean values of the gingival blood flow (GBF) recorded at various time points; interval plot of the four time points when the LDF measurements were carried out

$(SD = 74.9411)$; A: (a) sites with gingivitis; (b) healthy gingival site; B: restored gingival health after 14 days

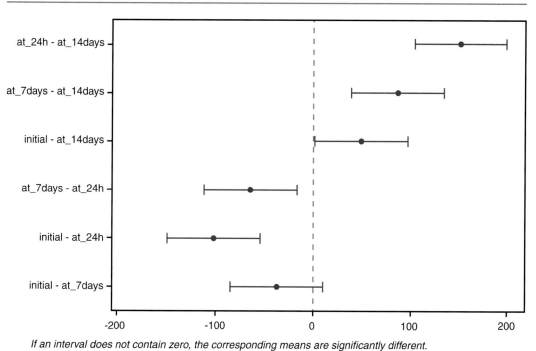

If an interval does not contain zero, the corresponding means are significantly different.

Fig. 4 Fisher individual 95% CIs. Comparison of GBF values of the gingivitis group at the four time points recorded in the study. No statistically significant differences were identified between the initial and the 7-day groups as well as between the initial and the 14-day groups

(LDR) and traditional clinical diagnostic indices as well as to evaluate the response to root planing in terms of LDR and traditional indices. LDR and clinical measurements (bleeding on probing (BOP), probing depth (PD), and clinical attachment loss (CAL)) were obtained from two healthy and two diseased sites in 30 adult volunteers with localized moderate to advanced periodontitis. All 30 subjects were re-examined 1 month following root planing while 10 subjects were re-examined at approximately 1 year after treatment. Subject-adjusted correlations between pre-treatment LDR and PD as well as LDR and CAL were 0.74 and 0.71, respectively. One month following root planing, the diseased sites had undergone a significant reduction in LDR and PD with an accompanying gain in CAL. Prior to treatment, 95 of 120 sites (79%) agreed on an ordinal classification (high, low) for LDR and BOP. Mantel-Haenszel common odds ratios for agreement between LDR and BOP were 9.6 pre-treatment and 4.3 1 month after treatment. A slight rebound of all measurements was noted in a group of ten subjects followed for 1 year. It was concluded that the laser Doppler periodontal probe is an unbiased noninvasive method of monitoring the response to periodontal therapy.

Laser Periodontal Surgery and Gingival Recovery

When performing gingivoplasty by conventional methods, there are limitations regarding healing by secondary intention, postoperative bleeding, loss of keratinized gingiva, and the inability to treat the underlying osseous deformities, which leads to the inability to complete the treatment [59]. The use of laser technologies to overcome these limitations is under investigation.

LDF techniques were found to have excellent utility for identifying post-surgical gingival recovery [60–62]. In order to establish the efficiency of one laser in comparison with another, we used LDF to compare GBF after Er:YAG (Fotona Fidelis Plus II) and 980 nm diode laser (Diode Laser Smile Pro 980 Biolitec) gingivec-

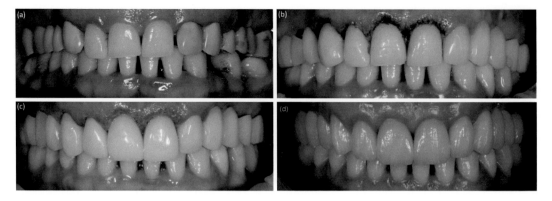

Fig. 5 (**a**) Initial intra-oral status, (**b**) immediately after laser surgery, (**c**) 24 h after the laser surgery with indirect provisional restorations, and (**d**) clinical intra-oral aspect 2 months after treatment with the final ceramic restorations

Fig. 6 The descriptive graphic for "Laser 1" method applied at the four timepoints

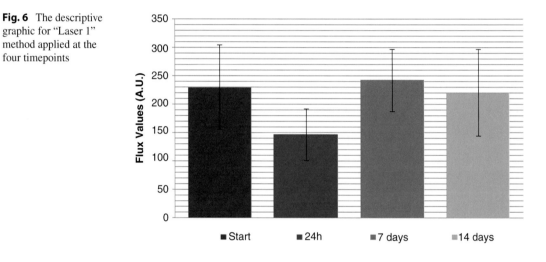

tomy. The evaluation was carried out on 20 anterior teeth that underwent reshaping of the gingiva in five patients (four anterior teeth/patient). The parameters were established according to previous research [26] and were found suitable for soft tissue without causing visible major thermal damage to root dentin or bone. The 980 nm diode laser was used in continuous wave mode, 4 W, contact mode, and cooling with saline solution using a 360 μm diameter quartz fiber as delivery system (Fig. 5) Er:YAG parameters.

At the first appointment, the initial measurements were carried out. Postoperative controls and LDF measurements were accomplished after 24 h, 7 and 14 days to evaluate healing and wound evolution on a total of eight points/patient (two points on each tooth). As for the gingival surgery

with Er:YAG laser, significant differences in LDF recordings over time were established between different times ($p < 0.001$ with a significant level $\alpha = 0.001$, Friedman test). The results showed that after 24 h there are significant differences compared to the baseline measurement; 7 days after treatment, with the Er:YAG, LDF was slightly raised compared to the initial moment ($p = 0.256$), and after 14 days, LDF values were insignificantly lower compared to pre-treatment ($p = 0.431$) (Fig. 6).

Regarding gingival surgery with the diode laser, significant differences between the four LDF tracings at different timepoints were found ($p < 0.001$ with a significant level $\alpha = 0.001$, Friedman test). After 24 h, the measurements were significantly lower compared to the initial

Fig. 7 The descriptive graphic for "Laser 2" method applied at the four timepoints

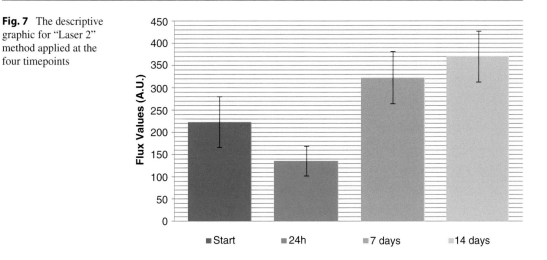

moment; whereas after 7 and 14 days, the recorded LDF values were significantly raised compared to baseline ($p < 0.001$) (Fig. 7).

The Levene's test for equality of variances was used in order to establish the equal variances assumed at baseline as well as after 14 days, and afterwards, the independent sample test was used for comparing the values obtained for the Er:YAG-treated area and for the diode-treated area at baseline (insignificant differences $p = 0.897$) and after 14 days (significant difference $p < 0.001$). We established that after 14 days, the recorded fluxes for the diode-treated area were significantly higher compared to the values obtained for the Er:YAG-treated area ($p < 0.001$).

The results obtained after laser treatment on the free gingival area indicate a modification in the microvascular blood flow response. Furthermore, our measurements, which are in accordance with other studies [33], indicate that LDF technique can offer information regarding microvascular changes during the healing period. These results showed an evident decrease in perfusion for both areas in comparison with baseline values 24 h after surgical procedure. The microvascular blood flow increased significantly after 7 days in both areas but mostly in the diode-treated area. After 14 days, the blood perfusion returned to the initial value in the Er:YAG-treated area. The results in the diode-treated area remained at a higher level, showing that after 14 days, the healing in this area was not complete.

The response after laser treatment in both areas was an obviously hyperemic one. The difference in hemodynamic changes that occurred after 14 days can be explained by the differences in tissue interaction of the different laser procedures applied in our study.

Smokers and Gingival Microcirculation

One of our studies [63] compared the periodontal status of smoker and non-smoker patients and also the registered values between the sexes (Fig. 8).

We found no significant differences (*t*-test) between the non-smoker male group (I-M) and non-smoker female group (I-F). On the other hand, LDF in the smoker female group (Group II-F) was significantly elevated compared to the smoker male group (Group II-M). The Group II-M LDF values were slightly increased compared to the Group I-M. The LDF values in the Group II-F were significantly higher than the LDF values in Group I-F.

Gingival Microcirculation Assessed by Laser Doppler Imaging

Essentially, laser Doppler imaging (LDI) works by scanning a monochromatic laser across the surface of the tissue. Light, which is backscattered from moving erythrocytes, undergoes a shift in frequency proportional to its velocity, according to the Doppler principle. Most laser Doppler setups use a helium-neon laser (RED, 632.8 nm), provide an estimate of perfusion to a

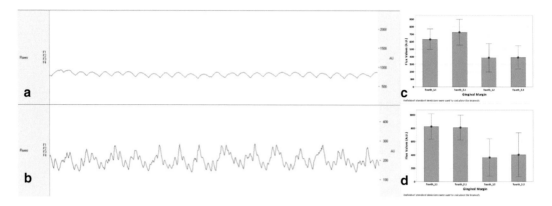

Fig. 8 (**a**) Example of LDF recording from a non-smoker patient; (**b**) example of LDF recording from a smoker patient; (**c**) interval plot of flux values (AU) in smoker male group; and (**d**) interval plot of flux values (A.U.) in smoker female group

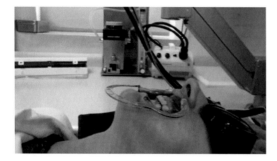

Fig. 9 Laser Doppler line scanning procedure

depth of 1–1.5 mm into the dermis of white skin, and thus mainly measure the perfusion in arterioles, venules, and capillaries. LDI gives a "snapshot" of perfusion at a given point.

The objective of one of our studies [64] was to evaluate the applicability of LD line scanning in recording the gingival healing process after a surgical procedure followed by two types of plastic provisional restoration. As a secondary objective, we also aimed at testing two different techniques and materials for the plastic temporaries. Conventional clinical examination was also performed at all time points.

The moorLDI2-IR instrument, features an infrared diode laser at 785 nm nominal, with a maximum power of 2.5 mW and a visible diode laser (target beam for infrared systems) at 660 nm nominal, with a maximum power of 0.25 mW, was used in our study. The microcirculation in the investigated areas was monitored with the Moor laser Doppler line scanner over a period of 14 days (Fig. 9).

LDI recordings were performed in the labial regions of the operated areas at the day of the surgery, prior to local anesthesia, after 24 h, after 7 days and 14 days following the intervention. The recordings clearly demonstrated adjustments in the microvascularity of the region in the healing period. The initial images (Fig. 10a) showed a perfusion map that differed completely from the LDI images at 24 h with increased microcirculation as a reaction to the surgical procedure (Fig. 10b), seen as an increase in the red color of the affected areas in the perfusion map. The LDI images on Day 7 showed microcirculation healing, while at 14 days complete healing was confirmed on the perfusion map. Clinical findings paralleled the perfusion maps in both cases. Using LDI, we were also able to demonstrate that two differing temporary restoration materials did not negatively affect healing.

The major advantages of LDI over LDF are: no need for direct tissue contact (max. distance 19 cm), measurement repeatability, and most importantly, the capability for global analysis of blood flow in the area of interest. This technique has been shown to be easy to learn by surgeons. Regular postoperative assessment of flap perfusion by members of the microsurgery team trained in the use of LD line scanning may, therefore, represent a practical alternative to more complex and invasive monitoring techniques. Issues of inter-

Fig. 10 (**a**) Initial LDI recording and (**b**) LDI recording at 24 h with an increase in the red color of the affected areas in the perfusion map

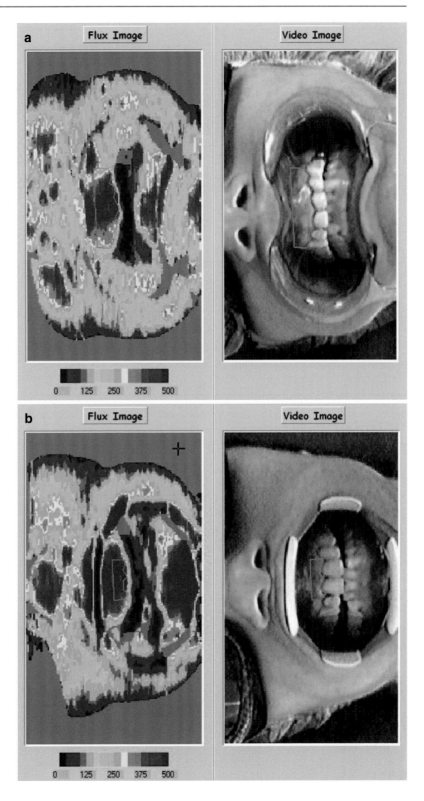

and intra-examiner reliability have yet to be examined, and in an area where only a low percentage of flaps undergo vascular compromise, this may prove impractical. One advantage that LDF has over LDI is that it gives a constant measure of blood flow at the specified point, whereas LDI gives a "snapshot" of perfusion at a given point.

Optical Coherence Tomography

Optical coherence tomography (OCT) is a noninvasive method of imaging dental microstructure which can potentially be used to evaluate the health of periodontal tissue. This method provides an "optical biopsy" of tissue 2–3 mm in depth. Optical coherence tomography was first proposed for use as a biologic imaging system in 1991 by Huang et al. In vivo dental OCT images clearly depict anatomic structures that are important in the diagnostic evaluation of both hard and soft oral tissue. Periodontal tissue contour, sulcular depth, and connective tissue attachment are visualized at high resolution using this technology. Because OCT reveals micro-structural detail of the periodontal soft tissues, it can potentially identify active periodontal disease before significant alveolar bone loss occurs.

Optical coherence tomography is potentially a more reproducible and reliable method of determining attachment level than traditional probing methods. The tissue of interest is imaged without making contact using a probe designed to have a focal plane at a distance from the probe tip. The tissues within the depth of field of the probe optics are imaged. A non-contact probe does not compress soft tissue and enables the direct geometric measurement of the dimensions of tissue in its natural state. In addition, an OCT probe may be designed with a short focus distance for direct contact imaging, allowing a sub-millimeter probe to be placed on the tissue surface or even in the pocket space.

The literature suggests that OCT is a powerful method for generating high-resolution, cross-sectional images of oral structures. However, further research is required to verify its role in periodontal diagnosis.

Assessment of Periodontal Structures and Measurement of Gingival Sulcus

There has been increasing interest in the development of clinically acceptable, more sensitive and specific methods for noninvasive diagnosis in periodontics. In a recent pilot study [65], the performance of an optical coherence tomography (OCT) system in imaging periodontal structures in humans was evaluated. Gingival sulcus depth measurements were obtained and compared with traditional probes. In total, 445 sites of 23 periodontally healthy individuals were measured by three instruments: North Carolina manual probe, Florida automated probe and OCT at 1325 nm. To obtain quantitative measurements from OCT images, the gingival refractive index was also determined. Discomfort/pain perception and the duration of examinations were compared among the instruments. The analysis of OCT images allowed the identification of relevant anatomic dental and periodontal regions. The average sulcus depth measured by OCT, 0.85 ± 0.27 mm and 0.87 ± 0.28 mm, was lower than the values obtained by manual and automated probing. Greater discomfort/pain was prevalent for traditional probes, which are invasive methods, than for the noninvasive OCT technique.

Calculus Detection

The effective treatment of periodontitis involves the detection and removal of sub-gingival dental calculus. However, sub-gingival calculus is more difficult to detect than supra-gingival calculus because it is firmly attached to root surfaces within periodontal pockets. To achieve a smooth root surface, clinicians often remove excessive amounts of root structure because of decreased visibility. In addition, enamel pearl, a rare type of ectopic enamel formation on the root surface, can easily be confused with dental calculus in the sub-gingival environment. In a recent study [66], we developed a fiber-probe swept-source optical coherence tomography (SSO-CT) technique and combined it with the quantitative measurement of optical parameters [standard deviation (SD) of the optical coherence tomography (OCT) intensity] to differentiate sub-gingival calculus from sound enamel, including enamel pearls. Two-dimensional circumferential images were constructed by rotating the mini-probe (0.9 mm diameter) while acquiring image lines, and the adjacent lines in each rotation were stacked to generate a three-dimensional volume. In OCT images, compared to sound enamel and enamel pearls, dental calculus showed significant differences ($P < 0.001$) in SD values. Finally, the receiver operating characteristic curve had a high capacity (area under the curve = 0.934) for discriminating between healthy regions (including enamel pearl) and dental calculus.

Periodontal Probing

Periodontitis is a multifactorial and infectious disease that may result in significant debilitation. The aim of one study [67] was to evaluate two optical coherence tomography (OCT) systems operating at 930 and 1325 nm, respectively, for structural analysis of periodontal tissue in porcine jaws. Two- and three-dimensional OCT images of the tooth/gingiva interface were acquired, and measurements of the gingival structures obtained from five fresh porcine jaws that were subsequently fixed, sectioned, and viewed using stereomicroscopy. The swept-source system operating at 1325 nm showed a better performance than the 930-nm spectral domain OCT system, owing to a longer central wavelength that allows deeper tissue penetration.

Periodontal Ligament Under Orthodontic Tooth Movement

Structural variations of the periodontal ligament (PDL) induced by orthodontic forces have been evaluated by optical coherence tomography (OCT) and compared to images obtained by conventional radiography [68]. In one study, two orthodontic appliances were installed on the maxillary anterior teeth of rats. Constant distraction force magnitudes of 0, 5, 10, and 30 gf were applied to four respective rats over 5 days. Then the rats were sacrificed and the maxillaries extracted for X-ray and OCT imaging. PDL changes proportional to the applied force magnitude were clearly visible in the OCT images, which also showed that a constant orthodontic force of 30 gf had torn the PDL. These results

support the clinical dental application of OCT for monitoring PDL changes during orthodontic procedures. The real-time imaging capability of OCT, together with its high resolution, has the potential to help dentists with in vivo orthodontic treatments in human subjects as well.

Optical coherence tomography (OCT) is a diagnostic tool that can make near-histologic tomographic images without a biohazard. Due to its high resolution (average, 4 μ) and safety (using light as the source), it has been applied widely in medical fields to replace invasive biopsies. But the trials in dentistry have been restricted to mainly detecting dental caries and oral cancer. In a preliminary study [69], we tried to evaluate whether OCT can be helpful in determining tooth movement under light orthodontic forces. Orthodontic distraction forces (0, 5, and 10 g) were applied to the mandibular incisors of six white rats (10 weeks old) for 5 days by using individualized loop springs (round Elgiloy, 0.018-in diameter, Rocky Mountain Orthodontics, Denver, Colo). The changed periodontal ligaments were imaged with OCT and digital intraoral radiography two dimensionally. Both tensile and compressive ligaments were measured and compared. With OCT images, we were able to measure changed ligaments from all directions; radiography could not show the portions overlapped by teeth. The averages of measured ligament width in OCT were larger than those from radiography in all groups. This preliminary study shows the possible evaluation and prediction of precise tooth responses under orthodontic forces by using real-time OCT.

Ultrasonic Flowmeters

By emitting and detecting reflected ultrasound, ultrasonic flow meters (UFM) [70] measure the velocity of a fluid and calculate its volume flow. The Doppler principle states that the frequency of the echo reflected from a moving target, such as red blood cells, will be different from the incident frequency [71]. Flow patterns can be detected by UFM from any accessible vessel, for instance, from the skin or oral mucosal surface. Ultrasound is sound with a frequency that is higher than 20 kHz. In medical imaging, utilized ultrasound frequencies mainly range between 1 and 40 MHz. The transmission through air of such high frequencies is impossible, but they can satisfactorily pass through solid or fluid materials [72].

Every flowmeter has a probe consisting of piezoelectric crystal, which generates the ultrasound beam. A second crystal, slightly separated from the first one, detects the reflected ultrasound. Thus every ultrasonic transducer has a dual function as a transmitter and receiver. The probe is applied to the skin, and a specialized ultrasonic gel is used to conduct ultrasound. A signal produced by an ultrasonic transducer usually consists of a pulse of a few microseconds with a certain center frequency. Part of this signal extends through the target tissue, part is reflected by macroscopic tissue structures, part is absorbed by tissue and part is scattered by structures in the tissue smaller than the acoustic wavelength. The ultrasound is translated into audible sound, which allows the operator to hear the pulsations in the vessel. Since the change in frequency is related to velocity, this can also be translated into vessel caliber. The UFM technique was originally proposed by Satomura, Matsubara, and Yoshioka (in 1956) for the physical measurement of minor vibrations [73]. In 1960, Satomura and Kaneko first described instantaneous changes in blood flow in human peripheral arteries using ultrasound blood-rheograph based on the Doppler Effect. Later, Strandness, McCutcheon, and Rushmer (in 1966) popularized transcutaneous flow detection for studying peripheral vascular problems [74].

The UFM technique in dentistry is a well-established diagnostic tool in Russia and some other countries. Several researchers have confirmed its usefulness for mapping periodontal lesions [75, 76].

The Doppler ultrasonic flowmeter has the following advantages:

1. Evaluation of blood in a limited gingival area (diameter of transducer is 1.5 mm)
2. Metal restorations are not a contraindication for use
3. Can interrogate pulpal blood flow

4. Possibility to detect blood flow in hard-to-access areas
5. Minimal time from measurement to results
6. Method is well tolerated by patients
7. Repeatable for monitoring uses

There are several standardization requirements for UFM:

1. Patient should be at rest; there should be no physical activity before use.
2. During measurements, patient should be reclining or sitting.
3. Comfortable room temperature (20–22 °C).
4. Refrain from smoking or chewing before measurements.
5. Investigator should not place pressure on the transducer.
6. During successive measurements, the transducer should be placed at the same position each time.

During ultrasonic blood flow investigation, the ultrasonic gel provides contact between the transducer and oral mucosa. A 20–25 MHz transducer is used to characterize periodontal blood flow. The ultrasound penetrates tissues to the depth of 0.8 cm. The transducer position can be controlled by sound and visual signals. The UFM can identify different types of blood vessels and distinguish between arterial, venous, and microcirculatory signals. The Doppler signal is processed and typically displayed as pulse curves with pseudo-color overlays called dopplerograms.

Dopplerograms help to visually determine the velocity of blood flow. It is known that the fastest erythrocytes are moving in the center of the blood vessel. On a dopplerogram, the fastest blood particles have a darker color and can be seen at the rim of the curve at a distance from the baseline, while the slowest blood particles are in the middle of the curve near the baseline. The direction of blood flow is also indicated: towards transducer ("+", upper part of the baseline) or away from transducer ("−", lower part of the baseline). Computer analysis of Doppler pulse curves provides information about the linear (systolic, mean, diastolic), and the volume velocity values of blood flow in the examined area. Qualitative and quantitative assessment of the blood flow is possible. The qualitative characteristic of the Doppler curve varies depending on the type and diameter of the vessel. Microcirculation (mixed blood flow) is characterized by pulse curves with a color spectrum that has no sharp peaks.

UFM has several advantages in comparison to Doppler laser flowmetry [77]:

1. Audible and visual control of the position of transducer
2. Ability to determine type of blood vessel by analyzing the blood flow curve
3. Ability to analyze differing flow speeds of specific blood vessel zones
4. Determination of blood flow direction

Optical Spectroscopy

Infrared Spectroscopy

Infrared (IR) spectroscopy is used increasingly in biomedical settings. It can distinguish differences in the characteristics of diverse molecules by probing the vibrations of chemical bonds and can use these molecular and sub-molecular profiles to define and differentiate between diseased and healthy tissues. As covalent bonds vibrate, they absorb energy in the form of IR light. The wavelength of light absorbed depends on the nature of the covalent bond, the type of vibration, and the environment of the bond. The IR spectrum of a tissue sample can be regarded as the molecular fingerprint of the tissue. If this molecular fingerprint is modified by a disease process, IR spectroscopy can be used to detect and monitor this process [78].

The IR spectrum of gingival crevicular fluid (GCF) is a rich source of information regarding the oral cavity and associated inflammation. Analysis of the IR spectrum of GCF, unlike traditional biochemical analyses, measures the total contents of GCF and may prove to be a powerful diagnostic and prognostic tool in periodontal diseases.

Xiang et al. [79] used IR spectroscopy to characterize GCF from healthy gingivitis and periodontitis sites and identified periodontitis-specific molecular signatures that clearly demarcated healthy and diseased tissues and thus can be used to confirm clinical diagnoses. Even in unpro-cessed spectral data, subtle differences in spectral band intensity and positions arising from the three major components (i.e., lipid, protein, and DNA) were observed in GCF from healthy gingivitis and periodontitis groups. Infrared spectroscopy may also provide a qualitative diagnosis of periodontal inflammatory status. This might be achieved by using linear discriminant analysis (LDA) to correlate observed spectral differences in GCF from sites with inflammatory conditions (gingivitis and periodontitis) and GCF of normal healthy status.

Infrared spectroscopy has the potential to simultaneously monitor multiple disease markers, including cellular infiltration and collagen catabolism. It represents a simple, reagent-free, multidimensional tool with which to examine periodontal disease etiology using entirely unprocessed tissue sections. As well as being highly accurate, the technique is straightforward and requires minimal training of operators [80].

Near-Infrared Spectroscopy

Another novel, noninvasive optical modality currently under exploration for periodontal disease diagnosis is NIR spectroscopy. This type of spectroscopy can be used to monitor hemodynamic and edema-based markers of soft tissues of the oral cavity. The water bands in gingival tissues provide an index of tissue hydration and thus may represent a simple indicator of inflammation at specific periodontal sites. Optical spectroscopy additionally offers a noninvasive means of assessing the balance between tissue oxygen delivery and oxygen utilization. Relative concentrations of oxygenated hemoglobin (HbO_2) and deoxygenated hemoglobin (Hb) can be measured by fitting optical attenuation spectra to the known optical properties (extinction coefficients) of HbO_2 and Hb. Thus, optical spectroscopy provides a measure of the hemoglobin–oxygen saturation of tissues and the degree of tissue perfusion. Based on these principles, Liu et al. [81] used NIR spectroscopy to demonstrate that tissue oxygenation at periodontitis sites was significantly decreased ($P < 0.05$) compared with that in gingivitis and healthy controls. A study performed by Ge et al. supports previous findings that tissue oxygenation as measured by optical spectroscopy is significantly decreased in periodontitis and can simultaneously determine multiple inflammatory indices related to periodontal disease directly in gingival tissues in vivo [82].

As tissue oxygen saturation is not measurable clinically, optical spectroscopy can provide a further index of inflammation that may be useful to the periodontist. Consequently, an NIR intra-oral probe may be able to determine sites at which disease has not yet clinically progressed, but which already manifest a biochemically defined profile suggestive of pathogenic potential, such as the anaerobicity required to establish a pathogenic microflora. Thus, optical spectroscopy appears to be a promising complementary method to clinical examination.

Conclusions

The major advantage of the laser Doppler techniques is their noninvasiveness and their ability to measure tissue microcirculation flux as well as fast stimulus-induced changes in perfusion. The LDF represents an important instrument to assess gingival and pulpal microcirculation in the oral cavity. In this respect, it can map tooth vitality, including pulp revascularization earlier than traditional sensitivity tests, which can also add to inflammation in an already irritated tissue. LDF can be used to assess the degree and duration of inflammation or ischemic episodes, thereby identifying patients at risk for adverse reactions such as irreversible inflammation, avascular necrosis, and tissue loss. In conclusion, LDF is a suitable technique for determining tissue vitality in most clinical situations and can be used together with other indices to evaluate the marginal gingival health status.

Dental OCT is able to generate high-resolution cross-sectional images of the superficial portions of the periodontal structures. Future improvements in imaging depth and the development of an intra-oral sensor are likely to make OCT a useful technique for periodontal applications.

The emergence of these various new technologies will certainly increase understanding

of periodontal diseases, eventually resulting in the development of risk assessment tools that will support better predictions of disease events. A more accurate system of determining prognosis would allow a more specific allocation of expenditure, thus improving the appropriateness and quality of dental care by minimizing the under- and overutilization of therapeutic options. A new paradigm for periodontal diagnosis would ultimately improve the clinical management of patients with periodontal disease.

Traditional Methods Vs. Minimally Invasive New Imaging Methods

Periodontitis is a prevalent disorder that affects most of the global population. Although the mild form of disease is compatible with good oral health, severe manifestations may lead to tooth loss. The World Health Organization has reported that severe periodontitis is present in 5–15% of people worldwide [83]. Furthermore, epidemiologic studies have shown that periodontal infection may also have implications for systemic health, suggesting that periodontitis is associated with a major oral health burden [84].

Periodontal diagnosis provides the clinician with information on the type, severity, and location of periodontal disease. A periodontal examination is performed to detect clinical signs of pain and suppuration, the amount of observable plaque and calculus, probing depths (PDs), and the extent and pattern of loss of clinical attachment and bone. Traditional clinical investigation tools for routine periodontal examinations are periodontal probing and conventional radiography. In periodontal probing, a manual probe is placed between the soft tissue and tooth to evaluate the sub-gingival periodontal condition. The PD is measured as the depth of probe penetration from the gingival margin to the base of the pocket. However, periodontal probing is not only painful for the patient but also prone to diagnostic inaccuracy, primarily because it is performed without visual guidance. Errors in PD measurements may be caused by the presence of dental calculus and inconsistencies in the force of probe insertion, in the diameter of the probe tip, and in the anatomical tooth contours. Moreover, reliable outcomes require the clinician to be sufficiently well trained in the technique.

The information provided by intra-oral radiographs includes root length, root form, presence or absence of periapical lesions, dental calculus, root proximity, and remaining alveolar bone. Conventional radiographs have a tendency to underestimate the amount of bone loss. Sequentially obtained radiographs have been shown to reveal bony changes that are detectable by the naked eye only after 30–50% of the bone mineral has been absorbed [85]. This means that radiographs are not useful for identifying periodontal disease until after substantial bone loss has already occurred. On two-dimensional (2D) radiographs, it is impossible to detect the precise location of a bony defect if the defect is located on the buccal or lingual side. Additionally, radiographs require exposure to harmful ionizing radiation and provide no information about the state of the soft tissues. Cone-beam computed tomography is routinely implemented in dentistry for imaging soft and hard tissues, especially for the diagnosis of oral pathology and three-dimensional (3D) analysis of oro-facial structures. However, its common use for periodontal diagnosis is questionable due to its relatively low spatial resolution and the need to expose patients to relatively high levels of ionizing radiation. To the best of our knowledge, there is no device available for consistently quantifying or visualizing the oral soft tissues.

Optical coherence tomography (OCT) is a noninvasive diagnostic technique that detects mechanical interfaces based on differences in the reflection of light. OCT enables subsurface cross-sectional imaging with a resolution better than ten times that of typical ultrasound imaging systems. OCT was initially developed for imaging the transparent tissues of the eye, but continuing advancements in OCT technology have led to the widespread use of existing prototypes

in fields of gastroenterology, ophthalmology, dermatology, and dentistry. OCT is also advantageous in dentistry since this technology uses nonionizing near-infrared light that cannot harm patients. Other advantages such as depth-resolved imaging, rapid acquisition of data, and the capability to observe both hard and soft tissues have made it attractive for many applications. OCT imaging of dental and periodontal microstructures may be useful for quantitative and qualitative assessments of oral tissues. The findings of a recent study [86] indicate that OCT can be used as a noninvasive method for imaging tooth microstructure. Many current OCT prototype systems operate in the Fourier domain (FD). One advantage of FD-OCT over previous OCT systems is that it simultaneously provides high-speed and wide field imaging. Depending on the method of illumination, FD-OCT can be classified into spectral domain OCT and swept-source OCT (SS-OCT). A recent animal study used an SS-OCT prototype for imaging the periodontal tissues and assessed its accuracy in periodontal diagnosis. Pocket depth measurements from OCT images were a mean of 0.41 mm shallower than those made in histological sections from the same sites. The measurements were carried out in the buccal furcation area of the mandibular premolars. The imaging depth required to observe the gingival attachment is greater inside the furcation than in other areas, due to the horizontal component of the furcal concavity. The cross-sectional imaging depth of the OCT system used in this study was found to be insufficient for visualizing the sulcus anatomy within the furcation, which is probably the main reason for the discrepancy between the depth measurements made using OCT and histologically.

The imaging depth of OCT is determined by two main factors: the wavelength of the light source and the numerical aperture of the light-collecting optics. Otis et al. [87] showed that image quality could be improved by increasing imaging depth, and that penetration depth could be increased by increasing the center wavelength of the light source. Similar results were obtained in a recent study of the porcine jaw, in which the performance of SS-OCT at 1325 nm was better than that at 930 nm owing to the longer center wavelength that allowed deeper tissue penetration [88]. In highly scattering media such as biologic tissue, the intensity of coherent backscattered light decays exponentially with depth. Moreover, increasing the source intensity has only a small effect on the imaging depth of OCT since the scattering coefficient is independent of the source power. In contrast, increasing the wavelength significantly reduces the scattering coefficient for many biologic tissues, including enamel and gingiva, but potentially decreases the spatial resolution of OCT images. A larger numerical aperture also improves the imaging depth resolution since the reflected light is collected over a larger range of scattering angles. The OCT system used in the present study had a relatively long center wavelength of 1310 nm with a numerical aperture of 0.026. Further developments in dental OCT are needed to improve both the imaging depth and the imaging quality before it can be utilized in periodontal applications.

The periodontal tissue contour, dental calculus, and connective tissue attachment were visualized in high definition using OCT in this study. Such detailed visualization of biologic tissues could be very useful in several fields of dentistry [89]. This may allow the early detection of active periodontal disease or causative factors such as sub-gingival calculus, before significant alveolar bone loss occurs. The captured images could be stored as a permanent record for comparison with future periodontal examinations in order to detect changes in PDs or the inflammatory response at sites of interest. This would provide valuable information during both the diagnostic and maintenance phases of periodontal therapy for the detection of disease recurrence or sites where periodontal treatment has been ineffective.

OCT images allow measurement of gingival thickness, which is a predictor of the gingival phenotype. Although image sharpness is affected by axial resolution and signal-to-noise ratio, it is possible to discriminate between the epithelium and sub-epithelial connective tissue. Such information can be immensely valuable and have implications for the results of periodontal therapy, gingival augmentation procedures, root coverage, and implants in esthetic areas where the adequacy of the gingival thickness is paramount. Determining the thickness of the epithelial layer can be especially useful during the planing and execution of connective tissue grafting procedures since this could confirm the sufficiency of undermining of the epithelium at the graft site. Furthermore, bleeding at the donor site could be reduced if palatal vessels are visualized. Several existing methods for evaluating gingival thickness, such as injection needles, probe transparency, and visual inspection, cannot be considered reliable due to their subjective nature. The main advantage of OCT over these techniques is that it is a quantitative high-resolution imaging method that can be used in real time during clinical procedures.

Brezinski et al. [90] showed that the contrast between different adjacent tissue types is stronger when there is a greater difference in the water content within tissues. Thus sub-gingival calculus, which has a higher water content than the adjacent tooth surface, also has a higher signal intensity and contrast. We may assume that the presence of gingival crevicular fluid in an in vivo model would allow better visualization of the sulcular anatomy compared to the ex vivo model. Future studies involving humans should investigate different gingival biotypes or pathologic tissues in order to test the clinical performance of dental OCT.

Future Developments

Although LDF has proved valuable for a variety of clinical applications, there are some limitations to its use in oral medicine. A major drawback is that LDF can only detect red blood cell movement in a small volume of tissue (1 mm^3); thus, variables such as the number of vessels with active flow, changes in vessel diameter, and flow in individual micro-vessels cannot be analyzed. The small measuring area may also influence the reproducibility of the results as a minimal displacement of the optical probe would alter the target area [91]. LDF measurements are affected by motion artifacts, and oral LDFRs have demonstrated considerable intra- and interindividual variability [92, 93]. As the velocity of PBF in humans is very low, LDF devices modified for measuring slow blood flow are needed [87]. One of the most important limitations of LDF is that each patient presents uncalibrated blood flow readings because the measurement is influenced by the thickness of the connective tissue and local distribution of the vessels and also the recording site (free gingiva, interdental gingiva, attached gingiva, or alveolar mucosa) [94, 95]. Another limitation of LDF is that flow readings are affected by the scattering properties of the surrounding tissues. It has been reported that up to 80% of the LD blood flow signal recorded from an intact human pulp is of non-pulpal origin [10]. The same could be anticipated for LDF measurements performed on the gingiva. Originally, iontophoresis was used in conjunction with single-point LDF, as opposed to LDI systems, which measure perfusion over a larger area and produce a detailed perfusion map. Laser Doppler flowmetry typically measures within a small volume ($\sim$1 mm^3) and, as a result, has often suffered from poor reproducibility, mainly due to the spatial heterogeneity of tissue blood flow and movement artifacts [96–98], although reproducibility has been improved recently by the use of "integrated probes." These use multiple collecting fibers positioned in a ring around a central light delivery fiber, thus increasing the spatial resolution. However, LDI still provides a larger surface area measurement and should be the preferred choice in areas of tissues with high spatial variability, despite the significant difference in costs.

Optical coherence tomography (OCT) was first reported by Fujimoto et al. in 1991 [99]. OCT has been widely used in numerous clinical applications, including gastroenterology [100], ophthalmology [101], dermatology [102], and dentistry [103]. OCT is a noninvasive, nonradiative optical diagnostic tool based on interferometers. By using a low-coherence broadband near-infrared light source, it is possible to obtain excellent spatial resolution ($\sim$20 μm) and real-time images [104]. OCT was first applied in vitro in the human retina and in atherosclerotic plaque [105]. It is an optical imaging technique that enables cross-sectional imaging of microstruc-

tures of tissue in situ. OCT can provide an "optical biopsy" without the need for excision and processing of specimens as in conventional biopsy and histopathology. With ongoing improvements in optical specifications and system capabilities, OCT demonstrates great potential in research and clinical applications.

Over the past decade, many functional OCT systems, such as Doppler OCT (DOCT) [106], polarization-sensitive OCT (PS-OCT) [107], endoscopic OCT [108], and acoustic OCT [109], have been utilized for novel biomedical research applications. These functional systems provide not only structural images but also inform on specific optical characteristics, including blood flow velocity and tissue orientation. Deeper transmission depths have been reported in combination with fluorescence [110]. Indeed, such multimodality approaches can enhance the diagnostic performance of OCT.

The first in vitro OCT images of dental hard and soft tissues in a porcine model were reported in 1998 [111], soon followed by in vivo imaging of human dental tissues [112]. The oral cavity consists of three main parts: (1) hard tissue, including tooth and alveolar bone, (2) soft tissue, including mucosa and gingiva tissues, and (3) periodontal tissues [113]. Traditional caries diagnosis is based on examination using a dental explorer and radiographs. Periodontal disease is diagnosed clinically using periodontal probes and radiographs. The poor sensitivity and reliability of periodontal probing hinders effective monitoring of disease status, progression, and treatment response [114]. Radiography may be the most widespread adjunct diagnostic tool. However, it typically provides only two-dimensional images. Caries or bone structure on the buccal and lingual sides of teeth may not be visible due to the superimposition of structures. Radiation exposure from radiographic techniques is also a great concern. Furthermore, early detection of caries, periodontal disease, and oral cancer is quite difficult using conventional clinical examination or radiographs.

OCT may provide a solution to these problems. Dental OCT detects qualitative and quantitative morphological changes of dental hard and soft tissues in vivo. Furthermore, OCT can also be used for early diagnosis of dental diseases, including caries, periodontal disease, and oral cancer, because of the excellent spatial resolution. Three-dimensional imaging ability is another advantage of dental OCT. It helps clinicians to locate problems in soft and hard tissues more accurately and rapidly.

Periodontitis is one of the major chronic infectious diseases in the oral cavity. The prevalence of periodontitis is more than 50% among the population [115]. The WHO revealed that tooth loss resulting from severe periodontitis was found in 5–15% of most worldwide populations in 2003 [116]. Additionally, recent studies have identified compelling correlations between periodontitis and various systemic diseases [117, 118]. Colston et al. were the first group to apply OCT in the diagnosis of periodontal disease [119]. They compared in vitro images of dental and periodontal tissues from a young porcine model and with histological sections. Feldchtein et al. demonstrated visible but poorly differentiated epithelium and lamina propria of gingival mucosa in OCT images [120]. Baek et al. published OCT images of periodontal ligaments during orthodontic movement in the rat [69]. Hsieh et al. demonstrated sub-gingival calculus in vitro, which is important as it is a significant and often clinically undetected pathogenetic factor of periodontal disease. The refractive indices of enamel, dentin, cementum, and calculus were measured as 1.625 ± 0.024, 1.534 ± 0.029, 1.570 ± 0.021, and 2.097 ± 0.094, respectively. The refractive indices help clinicians to distinguish calculus from normal tissues rapidly and correctly. With the aid of OCT, early detection of periodontal disease and monitoring of periodontal treatment could be very helpful. Further technological advances are required to reduce the procedure time and promote evaluation of posterior oral regions.

Size, Cost, Logistics, and Level of Training

Several factors constrain the adoption of dental OCT in clinical practice. The first issue is the small size of the area imaged in an OCT scan. Usually measuring just a few mm², hundreds or thousands of images may be necessary to image an entire lesion. Second, the limited penetration depth also restricts clinical utility. Choosing a high-quality light source may be a solution, however, this will increase the cost of the OCT system. Optical spectroscopy appears to be a promising complementary method for periodontal diagnosis. It allows for the instant capture of spectra, does not require any consumables, and, once the equipment is in place, it is very inexpensive to operate. It also requires minimal training to obtain reliable and reproducible data.

View to the Future

Several factors affecting the intra-oral performance of OCT are undergoing considerable improvements. Wavelength choice should be optimized. Within the near-infrared window, the center wavelength determines the maximum depth of tissue penetration based on its scattering and absorption properties. When the wavelength is under 1000 nm, scattering is the main determinant because of the similar size of light and particles in tissue. This phenomenon is often analyzed by Mie scattering theory. The absorption effect increases after 1000 nm and reaches the maximum around 1400 nm. Water in tissue will decay the input of light energy strongly. Therefore, different wavelengths are employed depending on the nature of the target tissues. For example, an OCT system with 1550 nm center wavelength is good for hard tissue measurement but not suitable for soft tissue imaging because the input light will be absorbed by blood or water. In dental applications, a 1550 nm system is suitable for imaging hard tissue, such as enamel, dentin, and alveolar bone, but not ideal for mucosal or gingival imaging.

Target tissue composition and uniformity also affect imaging performance. Samples with rough surfaces or inhomogeneous composition show lower penetration depth and image contrast due to scattering effects. Another important factor is the index difference between the sample and its background. Mismatches in the refractive index of the different tissue components result in light loss from optical scattering. Conversely, materials with similar refractive indices will demonstrate a similar appearance in OCT images. For example, retinal layers are difficult to distinguish because their similar composition translates into lack of contrast in OCT images. Functional OCT, including DOCT and PS-OCT, gathers more information in biological tissues. DOCT can inform on blood flow velocity and inflamed tissue volume. PS-OCT can inform on structural orientation.

For dental in vivo imaging, improved optical probe design—including probes for 3-D imaging—faster data acquisition and larger area scans are needed. OCT can obtain images in seconds. However, low image quality can result from faster imaging speeds due to insufficient processing time. Thus, equipment makers should optimize the balance between image quality and acquisition time. Because OCT imaging allows early detection of many oral diseases, including caries, periodontal disease, and oral cancer, future OCT systems should be telemedicine-compatible with a picture archiving and communication system (PACS). This will be helpful in home nursing care in our aging society and in low resource communities with limited access to dental care.

Laser and ultrasonic flowmeters can be valuable tools for periodontal diagnosis and management. They might be especially useful for predicting and preventing periodontal diseases as well as managing gingivitis and periodontitis. However, each approach provides different information about vascular events within a specific volume of tissue. Therefore, it is advisable to use them jointly to ensure accurate and detailed data for optimizing diagnosis and management of periodontal disease.

References

1. Sanz M, Newman MG, Quirynen M. Advanced diagnostic techniques. In: Newman MG, Takei HH, Klokkevold PR, Carranza FA, editors. Carranza's clinical periodontology. 10th ed. St Louis: Saunders; 2006. p. 579–601.
2. American Academy of Periodontology. Position paper: diagnosis of periodontal diseases. J Periodontol. 2003;74:1237–47.
3. Michaud DS, Liu Y, Meyer M, Giovannucci E, Joshipura K. Periodontal disease, tooth loss, and cancer risk in male health professionals: a prospective cohort study. Lancet Oncol. 2008;9:550–8.
4. Petersen PE, Bourgeois D, Ogawa H, Estupinan-Day S. Ndiaye: the global burden of oral diseases and risks to oral health. Bull World Health Organ. 2005;83:661–9.
5. Albandar JM, Brunelle JA, Kingman A. Destructive periodontal disease in adults 30 years of age and older in the United States, 1988–1994. J Periodontol. 1999;70:13–29. Erratum, 70:351.
6. Berezow AB, Darveau RP. Microbial shift and periodontitis. Periodontol 2000. 2011;55:36–47.
7. D'Aiuto F, Parkar M, Andreaou G, Brett PM, Ready D, Tonetti MS. Periodontitis and atherogenesis: causal association or simple coincidence? J Clin Periodontol. 2004;31:402–11.
8. De Backer D, Donadello K, Taccone FS, Ospina-Tascon G, Salgado D, Vincent JL. Microcirculatory alterations: potential mechanisms and implications for therapy. Ann Intensive Care. 2011;1:27.
9. Develioglu H, Kesim B, Tuncel A. Evaluation of the marginal gingival health using laser Doppler flowmetry. Braz Dent J. 2006;17:219–22.
10. Develioglu H, Ozcan G, Taner L, Ozgören O. A limited and useful approach to determine proximal periodontal health. West Indian Med J. 2010;59: 215–8.
11. Gleissner C, Kempski O, Peylo S, Glatxel JH, Willershausen B. Local gingival blood flow at healthy and inflamed sites measured by laser Doppler flowmetry. J Periodontol. 2006;77:1762–71.
12. Taba M, Kinney J, Kim AS, et al. Diagnostic biomarkers for oral and periodontal diseases. Dent Clin North Am. 2005;49:551–71.
13. Giannobile WV, Beikler T, Kinney JS, et al. Saliva as a diagnostic tool for periodontal disease: current state and future directions. Periodontol 2000. 2009;50:52–64.
14. Zhang L, Henson BS, Camargo PM, et al. The clinical value of salivary biomarkers for periodontal disease. Periodontol 2000. 2009;51:25–37.
15. Tenenbaum HC, Tenenbaum H, Zohar R. Future treatment and diagnostic strategies for periodontal diseases. Dent Clin North Am. 2005;49:677–94.
16. Stern MD. In vivo evaluation of microcirculation by coherent light scattering. Nature. 1975;254:56–8. https://doi.org/10.1038/254056a0.
17. Kerdvongbundit V, Sirirat M, Sirikulsathean A, Kasetsuwan J, Hasegawa A. Blood flow and human periodontal status. Odontology. 2002;90(1):52–6.
18. Hinrichs JE, LaBelle LL, Aeppli D. An evaluation of laser Doppler readings obtained from human gingival sulci. J Periodontol. 1995;66:171–6. https://doi.org/10.1902/jop.1995.66.3.171.
19. Kerdvongbundit V, Vongsavan N, Soo-Ampon S, Hasegawa A. Microcirculation and micromorphology of healthy and inflamed gingivae. Odontologia. 2003;91(1):19–25. https://doi.org/10.1007/s102660200007.

20. Kindlová M. The blood supply of the marginal periodontium in Macacus rhesus. Arch Oral Biol. 1965;10:869–74.
21. Egelberg J. The blood vessels of the dento-gingival junction. J Periodontal Res. 1966;1:163–79.
22. Hansson BO, Lindhe J, Branemark PI. Microvascular topography and function in clinically healthy and chronically inflamed dentogingival tissues—a vital microscopic study in dogs. Periodontics. 1968;6:264–71.
23. Hock J, Nuki K. A vital microscopy study of the morphology of normal and inflamed gingiva. J Periodontal Res. 1971;6:81–8. https://doi.org/10.1111/j.1600-0765.1971.tb00592.x.
24. Nuki K, Hock J. The organization of the gingival vasculature. J Periodontal Res. 1974;9:305–13. https://doi.org/10.1111/j.1600-0765.1974.tb00686.x.
25. Vág J, Fazekas A. Influence of restorative manipulations on the blood perfusion of human marginal gingiva as measured by laser Doppler flowmetry. J Oral Rehabil. 2002;29(1):52–7. https://doi.org/10.1046/j.1365-2842.2002.00818.x.
26. Hock J, Nuki K, Schlenker R, Hawks A. Clearance rates of Xenon-133 in non-inflamed and inflamed gingiva of dogs. Arch Oral Biol. 1980;25:445–9. https://doi.org/10.1016/0003-9969(80)90050-3.
27. Clarke NG, Shepherd BC, Hirsch RS. The effects of intra-arterial epinephrine and nicotine on gingival circulation. Oral Surg Oral Med Oral Pathol. 1981;52:577–82. https://doi.org/10.1016/0030-4220(81)90071-2.
28. Kaplan ML, Jeffcoat MK, Goldhaber P. Blood flow in gingiva and alveolar bone in beagles with periodontal disease. J Periodontal Res. 1982;17:384–9. https://doi.org/10.1111/j.1600-0765.1982.tb01169.x.
29. Akpinar KE, Er K, Polat S, Polat NT. Effect of gingiva on laser Doppler pulpal blood flow measurements. J Endod. 2004;30(3):138–40. https://doi.org/10.1097/00004770-200403000-00003.
30. Matsuo M, Okudera T, Takahashi SS, Wada-Takahashi S, Maeda S, Iimura A. Microcirculation alterations in experimentally induced gingivitis in dogs. Anat Sci Int. 2017;92:112–7. https://doi.org/10.1007/s12565-015-0324-8.
31. Keremi B, Csempesz F, Vag J, Gyorfi A, Fazekas A. Blood flow in marginal gingiva as measured with laser Doppler. Fogorv Sz. 2000;10:163–8.
32. Kerdvongbundit V, Vongsavan N, Soo-Ampon S, Phankosol P, Hasegawa A. Microcirculation of the healthy human gingiva. Odontology. 2002;90:48–51.
33. Donos N, D'Aiuto F, Retzepi M, Tonetti M. Evaluation of gingival blood flow by the use of laser Doppler flowmetry following periodontal surgery: a pilot study. J Periodontal Res. 2005;40:129–37.
34. Matheny JL, Jhonson DT, Vroth GI. Aging and microcirculatory dynamics in human gingiva. J Clin Periodontol. 1993;20:471–5.
35. Perry DA, Macdowell J, Goodis HI. Gingival microcirculation response to tooth brushing measured by laser Doppler flowmetry. J Periodontol. 1997;68:990–5.
36. Öberg PA, Hollaway G. Gingival blood flow measured with a laser Doppler flowmetry. J Periodontol. 1986;21:73–85.
37. Vag J, Fazekas A. Influence of restorative manipulations on the blood perfusion of human marginal gingiva as measured by laser Doppler flowmetry. J Oral Rehabil. 2002;29:52–7.
38. al-Wahadni A, Linden GJ, Hussey DL. Periodontal response to cantilevered and fixed-fixed resin bonded bridges. Eur J Prosthodont Restor Dent. 1999;7:57–60.
39. Baab DA, Oberg A, Lundstrom A. Gingival blood flow and temperature changes in young humans with a history of periodontitis. Arch Oral Biol. 1990;35:95–101.
40. Hock JM, Kim S. Blood flow in healed and inflamed tissue of dogs. J Periodontal Res. 1987;22:1–5.
41. Wilder-Smith P, Frosch P. Laser Doppler flowmetry: a method for the determination of periodontal blood flow. Dtsch Zahnarztl Z. 1988;43:994–7.
42. Kerdvongbundit V, Vongsavan N, Soo-Ampon S, Hasegawa A. Microcirculation and micromorphology of healthy and inflamed gingivae. Odontology. 2003;91:19–25.
43. Matheny JL, Abrams H, Johnson DT, Roth GI. Microcirculatory dynamics in experimental human gingivitis. J Clin Periodontol. 1993;20:578–83.
44. Baab DA, Oberg PA. Laser Doppler measurement of gingival blood flow in dogs with increasing and decreasing inflammation. Arch Oral Biol. 1987;32:551–5.
45. Hinrichs JE, Jarzembinski C, Hardie N, Aeppli D. Intrasulcular laser Doppler readings before and after root planing. J Clin Periodontol. 1995;22:817–23.
46. Retzepi M, Tonetti M, Donos N. Gingival blood flow changes following periodontal access flap surgery using laser Doppler flowmetry. J Clin Periodontol. 2007;34:437–43.
47. Retzepi M, Tonetti M, Donos N. Comparison of gingival blood flow during healing of simplified papilla preservation and modified Widman flap surgery: a clinical trial using laser Doppler flowmetry. J Clin Periodontol. 2007;34:903–11.
48. Baab DA, Oberg PA. The effect of cigarette smoking on gingival blood flow in humans. J Clin Periodontol. 1987;14:418–24.
49. Mavropoulos A, Aars H, Brodin P. Hyperaemic response to cigarette smoking in healthy gingiva. J Clin Periodontol. 2003;30:214–21.
50. Palmer RM, Scott DA, Meekin TN, Poston RN, Odell EW, Wilson RF. Potential mechanisms of susceptibility to periodontitis in tobacco smokers. J Periodontal Res. 1999;34:363–9.

51. Mullally BH. The influence of tobacco smoking on the onset of periodontitis in young persons. Tob Induc Dis. 2004;2:6.

52. Meekin TN, Wilson RF, Scott DA, Ide M, Palmer RM. Laser Doppler flowmeter measurement of relative gingival and forehead skin blood flow in light and heavy smokers during and after smoking. J Clin Periodontol. 2000;27:236–42.

53. Ketabi M, Hirsch RS. The effects of local anesthetic containing adrenaline on gingival blood flow in smokers and non-smokers. J Clin Periodontol. 1997;24:888–92.

54. Yamaguchi K, Nanda RS, Kawata T. Effect of orthodontic forces on blood flow in human gingiva. Angle Orthod. 1991;61:193–204.

55. Yamaguchi K, Nanda RS. Blood flow changes in gingival tissues due to the displacement of teeth. Angle Orthod. 1992;62:257–64.

56. Barta A, Nagy G, Csiki Z, Márton S, Madléna M. Changes in gingival blood flow during orthodontic treatment. Cent Eur J Med. 2010;5:758–65.

57. Canjau S, Miron MI, Todea CD. Laser Doppler flowmetry evaluation of gingival microcirculation recovery in gingivitis. Arch Balkan Med Union. 2015;50(3):354–9.

58. Ramsay DS, Artun J, Martinen SS. Reliability of pulpal blood-flow measurements utilizing laser Doppler flowmetry. J Dent Res. 1991;70:1427–30. https://doi.org/10.1177/00220345910700110601.

59. Cohen ES. Atlas of cosmetic and reconstructive periodontal surgery. 3rd ed. Hamilton: BC Decker Inc.; 2007.

60. Ishikawa I, Aoki A, Takasaki AA. Potential applications of erbium: YAG laser in periodontics. J Periodontal Res. 2004;39:275–85. https://doi.org/10.1111/j.1600-0765.2004.00738.x.

61. Walsh LJ. The current status of laser applications in dentistry. Aust Dent J. 2003;48(3):146–55. https://doi.org/10.1111/j.1834-7819.2003.tb00025.x.

62. Kenneth S, Magid R, Strauss A. Laser use for esthetic soft tissue modification. Dent Clin North Am. 2007;51:525–45. https://doi.org/10.1016/j.cden.2006.12.005.

63. Vitez B, Todea C, Velescu A, Şipoş C. Evaluation of gingival vascularisation using laser Doppler flowmetry. Proc. SPIE 9670, sixth international conference on lasers in medicine, 96700J. 2016. https://doi.org/10.1117/12.2191859.

64. Noditi G, Todea C. Laser Doppler imaging—as a non-invasive method for assessing regional microcirculation when using plastic materials for guided healing. Mater Plast. 2013;1(50):40–3.

65. Fernandes LO, Mota CC, de Melo LS, da Costa Soares MU, da Silva Feitosa D, Gomes AS. In vivo assessment of periodontal structures and measurement of gingival sulcus with optical coherence tomography: a pilot study. J Biophotonics. 2016;10:862. https://doi.org/10.1002/jbio.201600082. [Epub ahead of print]

66. Kao MC, Lin CL, Kung CY, Huang YF, Kuo WC. Miniature endoscopic optical coherence tomography for calculus detection. Appl Opt. 2015;54(24):7419–23.

67. Mota CC, Fernandes LO, Cimões R, Gomes AS. Non-invasive periodontal probing through Fourier-domain optical coherence tomography. J Periodontol. 2015 Sep;86(9):1087–94.

68. Na J, Lee BH, Baek JH, Choi ES. Optical approach for monitoring the periodontal ligament changes induced by orthodontic forces around maxillary anterior teeth of white rats. Med Biol Eng Comput. 2008;46(6):597–603.

69. Baek JH, Na J, Lee BH, Choi E, Son WS. Optical approach to the periodontal ligament under orthodontic tooth movement: a preliminary study with optical coherence tomography. Am J Orthod Dentofac Orthop. 2009;135(2):252–9.

70. Kaplan EN, Vistnes LM. The Doppler flow meter. Calif Med. 1972;116:57–8.

71. Atkinson P, Wells PN. Pulse-Doppler ultrasound and its clinical application. Yale J Biol Med. 1977;50:367–73.

72. Postema M, Gilja OH. Contrast-enhanced and targeted ultrasound. World J Gastroenterol. 2011;17:28–41.

73. Nimura Y, Matsuo H, Hayashi T, Kitabatake A, Mochizuki S. Studies on arterial flow patterns—instantaneous velocity spectrums and their phasic changes—with directional ultrasonic Doppler technique. Br Heart J. 1974;36:899–907.

74. Al Turk M, Metcalf WK. A study of superficial palmar arteries using the Doppler ultrasonic flowmeter. J Anat. 1984;138:27–32.

75. Musaeva R, Barmasheva A, Orekchova L. Periodontal condition and microcirculation in patients with different number of metabolic syndrome components [abstract]. J Clin Periodontol. 2012;39.(Suppl. 13s:115.

76. Krechina EK, Belorukov VV. Artemisia absinthium L. in complex treatment of inflammatory periodontal disease. Stomatologiia (Mosk). 2012;91:22–4. (Russian)

77. Kozlov VA, Artyushenko NK, Shalack OV, Vasiliev AV, Girina MB, Girin II, Morozova EA, Monastirenko AA. Dopplerografiya v ocenke sostoyaniya gemodynamici v tkanyax shei, lica I polosti rta v norme i pri nekotorix patologicheskix sostoyaniyax. St. Petersburg: Medicinskaya Akademiya poslediplomnogo obrazovaniya; 2000. p. 31.

78. Hynes A, Scott DA, Man A, et al. Molecular mapping of periodontal tissues using infrared microspectroscopy. BMC Med Imaging. 2005;5:2.

79. Xiang XM, Liu KZ, Man A, et al. Periodontitis-specific molecular signatures in gingival crevicular fluid. J Periodontal Res. 2010;45:345–52.

80. Xiang X, Sowa MG, Iacopino AM, et al. Review: an update on novel non-invasive approaches for periodontal diagnosis. J Periodontol. 2010;81:186–98.

81. Liu KZ, Xiang XM, Man A, et al. In vivo determination of multiple indices of periodontal inflammation by optical spectroscopy. J Periodontal Res. 2009;44:117–24.

82. Ge Z, Liu KZ, Xiang X, et al. Assessment of local haemodynamics in periodontal inflammation using optical spectroscopy. J Periodontol. 2011;82:1161–8.

83. Burt B, Research, Science and Therapy Committee of the American Academy of Periodontology. Position paper: epidemiology of periodontal diseases. J Periodontol. 2005;76:1406–19.

84. Petersen PE, Ogawa H. The global burden of periodontal disease: towards integration with chronic disease prevention and control. Periodontol 2000. 2012;60:15–39.

85. Je coat MK, Wang IC, Reddy MS. Radiographic diagnosis in periodontics. Periodontol 2000. 1995;7:54–68.

86. Park J-Y, Chung J-H, Lee J-S, Kim H-J, Choi S-H, Jung U-W. Comparisons of the diagnostic accuracies of optical coherence tomography, micro-computed tomography, and histology in periodontal disease: an ex vivo study. J Periodontal Implant Sci. 2017;47(1):30–40.

87. Otis LL, Colston BW Jr, Everett MJ, Nathel H. Dental optical coherence tomography: a comparison of two in vitro systems. Dentomaxillofac Radiol. 2000;29:85–9.

88. Mota CC, Fernandes LO, Cimões R, Gomes AS. Non-invasive periodontal probing through fourier- domain optical coherence tomography. J Periodontol. 2015;86:1087–94.

89. Canjau S, Todea C, Negrutiu ML, Sinescu C, Topala FI, Marcauteanu C, Manescu A, Duma V-F, Bradu A, Podoleanu AGH. Optical coherence tomography for non-invasive ex vivo investigations in dental medicine—a joint group experience (review). Sovremennye tehnologii v medicine. 2015;7(1):97–115.

90. Brezinski ME, Tearney GJ, Bouma BE, Izatt JA, Hee MR, Swanson EA, et al. Optical coherence tomography for optical biopsy. Properties and demonstration of vascular pathology. Circulation. 1996;93:1206–13.

91. Boutault F, Cadenat H, Hibert PJ. Evaluation of gingival microcirculation by a laser-Doppler flowmeter. J Craniomaxillofac Surg. 1989;17:105–9.

92. Hoke JA, Burkes EJ, White JT, Duffy MB, Klitzman B. Blood-flow mapping of oral tissues by laser Doppler flowmetry. Int J Oral Maxillofac Surg. 1994;23:312–5.

93. Sasano T, Shoji N, Kuriwada S, Sanjo D. Calibration of laser Doppler flowmetry for measurement of gingival blood flow. J Periodontal Res. 1995;30:298–301. https://doi.org/10.1111/j.1600-0765.1995.tb02138.x.

94. Karayilmaz H, Kirzioglu Z. Comparison of the reliability of laser Doppler flowmetry, pulse oximetry and electric pulp tester in assessing the pulp vitality of human teeth. J Oral Rehabil. 2011;38(5):340–7. https://doi.org/10.1111/j.1365-284of2.2010.02160.x.

95. Miron MI, Dodenciu D, Saarbescu PF, Filip LM, Balabuc CA, Hanigovski E, Todea DC. Optimization of the laser Doppler signal acquisition technique in pulp vitality tests. Arch Balkan Med Union. 2011;46(4):280–4.

96. Morris SJ, Shore AC. Skin blood flow responses to the iontophorosis of acetylcholine and sodium nitroprusside in man: possible mechanisms. J Physiol. 1996;496:531–42. https://doi.org/10.1113/jphysiol.1996.sp021704.

97. Bonner R, Nossal R. Model for laser Doppler measurements of blood flow in tissue. Appl Opt. 1981;20:2097–107. https://doi.org/10.1364/AO.20.002097.

98. Tew GA, Klonizakis M, Crank H, Briers JD, Hodges GJ. Comparison of laser speckle contrast imaging with laser Doppler for assessing microvascular function. Microvasc Res. 2011;82:326–32. https://doi.org/10.1016/j.mvr.2011.07.007.

99. Huang D, Swanson EA, Lin CP, Schuman JS, Stinson WG, Chang W, Hee MR, Flotte T, Gregory K, Puliafito CA, Fujimoto JG. Optical coherence tomography. Science. 1991;254:1178–81.

100. Smith PW, Lee K, Guo S, Zhang J, Osann K, Chen Z, Messadi D. In vivo diagnosis of oral dysplasia and malignancy using optical coherence tomography: preliminary studies in 50 patients. Lasers Surg Med. 2009;41:353–7.

101. Wang Y, Bower BA, Izatt JA, Tan O, Huang D. Retinalblood flow measurement by circumpapillary Fourier domain Doppler optical coherence tomography. J Biomed Opt. 2008;13:064003. https://doi.org/10.1117/1.2998480.

102. Pierce MC, Strasswimmer J, Park BH, Cense B, de Boer JF. Birefringence measurements in human skin using polarization-sensitive optical coherence tomography. J Biomed Opt. 2004;9:287–91.

103. Clarkson DM. An update on optical coherence tomography in dentistry. Dent Update. 2014;41(2):174–6, 179–80.

104. Wojtkowski M, Srinivasan V, Fujimoto JG, Ko T, Schuman JS, Kowalczyk A, Duker JS. Three-dimensional retinal imaging with high-speed ultrahigh-resolution optical coherence tomography. Ophthalmology. 2005;112:1734–46.

105. Brezinski ME, Tearney GJ, Weissman NJ, Boppart SA, Bouma BE, Hee MR, Weyman AE, Swanson EA, Southern JF, Fujimoto JG. Assessing atherosclerotic plaque morphology: comparison of optical coherence tomography and high frequency intravascular ultrasound. Heart. 1997;77:397–403.

106. Yang XDV, Mao YX, Munce N, Standish B, Kucharczyk W, Marcon NE, Wilson BC, Vitkin IA. Interstitial Doppler optical coherence tomography. Opt Lett. 2005;30:1791–3.

107. Pircher M, Goetzinger E, Leitgeb R, Hitzenberger C. Three dimensional polarization sensitive OCT of human skin in vivo. Opt Express. 2004;12:3236–44.

108. Pan YT, Xie HK, Fedder GK. Endoscopic optical coherence tomography based on a microelectrome-chanical mirror. Opt Lett. 2010;26:1966–8.

109. Lesaffre M, Farahi S, Boccara AC, Ramaz F, Gross M. Theoretical study of acousto-optical coherence tomography using random phase jumps on ultrasound and light. J Opt Soc Am A. 2011;28:1436–44.

110. Iftimia N, Iyer AK, Hammer DX, Lue N, Mujat M, Pitman M, Ferguson RD, Amiji M. Fluorescence-guided optical coherence tomography imaging for colon cancer screening: a preliminary mouse study. Biomed Opt Express. 2012;3:178–91.

111. Colston BW, Everett MJ Jr, da Silva LB, Otis LL, Stroeve P, Nathel H. Imaging of hard- and soft-tissue structure in the oral cavity by optical coherence tomography. Appl Opt. 1998;37:3582–5.

112. Drexler W, Fujimoto JG. Optical coherence tomography: technology and applications. Berlin: Springer; 2008.

113. Hsieh YS, Ho YC, Lee SY, Lu CE, Jiang CP, Chuang CC, Wang CY, Sun CW. Subgingival calculus imaging based on swept-source optical coherence tomography. J Biomed Opt. 2011;16:071409. https://doi.org/10.1117/1.3602851.

114. Xiang X, Sowa MG, Iacopino AM, Maev RG, Hewko MD, Man A, Liu KZ. An update on novel non-invasive approaches for periodontal diagnosis. J Periodontol. 2009;81:186–98.

115. Hugoson A, Sjödin B, Norderyd O. Trends over 30 years, 1973-2003, in the prevalence and severity of periodontal disease. J Clin Periodontol. 2008;35:405–14.

116. Petersen PE. The world oral health report. Geneva: World Health Organization; 2003.

117. Khader YS, Ta'ani Q. Periodontal diseases and the risk of preterm birth and low birth weight: a meta-analysis. J Periodontol. 2005;76:161–5.

118. Beck JD, Offenbach S. Systemic effects of periodontitis: epidemiology of periodontal disease and cardiovascular disease. J Periodontol. 2005;76(11-s):2089–100.

119. Colston BW, Everett MJ, Silva LBD, Otis LL, Nathel H. Optical coherence tomography for diagnosing periodontal disease. Proc SPIE. 1997;2973:216–20.

120. Feldchtein F, Gelikonov V, Iksanov R, Gelikonov G, Kuranov R, Sergeev A, Gladkova N, Ourutina M, Reitze D, Warren J. In vivo OCT imaging of hard and soft tissue of the oral cavity. Opt Express. 1998;3:239–50.

Imaging Oral Biofilm and Plaque

Janet Ajdaharian and Jae Ho Baek

Abstract

Oral biofilm is a primary determinant of oral health, yet our ability to detect, map, and characterize it in vivo remains extremely limited. Moreover, there exists an as yet unmet but pressing need for characterizing its properties and response to prevention and intervention measures. Because clinical mapping of oral biofilm has been primarily restricted to macroscopic plaque staining techniques combined with naked eye visualization, additional means of assessing and quantifying oral biofilm in situ at high levels of resolution are currently under development. This chapter addresses emerging optical imaging modalities for evaluating in vivo oral biofilm noninvasively. Desirable attributes include: informing on variables that translate into clinical decision-making guidance to improve diagnosis, better treatment planning and outcomes, ease and speed of use, appropriate cost for the indicated setting, patient-friendly probes, and reliability. In this chapter, the principles behind optical approaches to imaging and characterizing oral biofilm, as well as their feasibility and applicability for imaging in situ are reviewed.

J. Ajdaharian
Beckman Laser Institute, University of California, Irvine, CA, USA

J. H. Baek (✉)
Department of Orthodontics, Dental Hospital, Pusan National University, Yangsan City, South Korea

Department of Dentistry, Ulsan University Hospital, Ulsan City, South Korea

WeSmile Orthodontic Clinic, Ulsan City, South Korea

© Springer Nature Switzerland AG 2020
P. Wilder-Smith, J. Ajdaharian (eds.), *Oral Diagnosis*, https://doi.org/10.1007/978-3-030-19250-1_4

Background

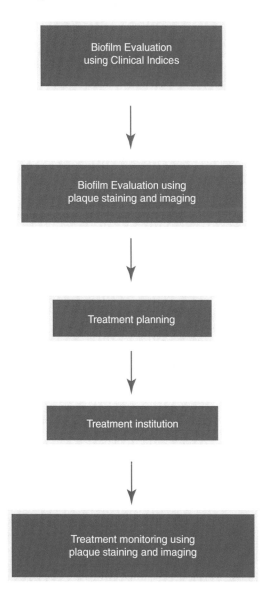

Biofilm Evaluation using Clinical Indices

Biofilm Evaluation using plaque staining and imaging

Treatment planning

Treatment institution

Treatment monitoring using plaque staining and imaging

Biofilm affects all aspects of our daily lives and is seminal in establishing, maintaining, and evaluating oral health [1]. Oral biofilm is typically referred to as dental plaque. It colonizes oral structures rapidly, and its thickness increases slowly with time. Although the literature reports a wide range of values, typically its thickness would approximate 20–30 μm after 3 days [2]. Initially, selective adsorption of salivary biopolymers on the enamel surface leads to the formation of the acquired salivary pellicle [3]. The adsorbed layer is a dynamic biofilm that can affect interactions at the interface between tooth surface and oral cavity [3–7]. Much research has been reported on the potential health hazards posed by biofilm [8], and microbial biofilms are implicated in the etiopathogenesis of many oral conditions including caries and periodontal disease [2]. Biofilms can have undesirable effects, for example, when they colonize medical and dental implants, but they can also be harnessed for beneficial purposes, such as when they are used for waste treatment [9]. Oral biofilm contains a multitude of factors important to oral microbial ecology and tissue surface properties. For example, the morphology of the oral biofilm layer appears to affect bacterial binding to the tooth surface [10, 11]. Because of this ambiguity and complexity of oral biofilm, understanding oral biofilm correctly is an essential process to reveal and prevent oral diseases (Table 1).

The first rudimentary characterization of dental plaque or biofilm was performed by van Leeuwenhoek with a microscope in 1683 [12]. However, despite enormous technological advances since that time, our ability to evaluate oral plaque accurately remains very limited due to the instability of the oral biofilm and the physical limitations on the use of microscopes within the oral cavity. It is only the recent development of miniaturized, multimodal high-resolution imaging technology that has begun to permit intra-oral analysis of oral biofilm (Table 2).

Table 1 Overview of chapter content: techniques for oral diagnosis

Existing techniques	Available minimally invasive methods	New imaging methods
Clinical examination; Clinical indices; Plaque staining	Plaque staining combined with image analysis techniques; Confocal laser scanning microscopy; Atomic force microscopy	Optical coherence tomography; Optical coherence microscopy; Multiphoton microscopy; Light sheet fluorescence microscopy

Table 2 Conventional imaging approaches for oral biofilm

Technology	Advantages	Disadvantages
Confocal laser scanning microscopy (CLSM)	Very high resolution (1 µm)	Limited imaging depth (100 µm) Photo damage to sample
Multiphoton fluorescence microscopy (MPM)	Greater imaging depth than CLSM (>100 µm)	Photo damage over threshold
Atomic force microscopy (AFM)	Ultra-high atomic level resolution	Surface imaging only
Light sheet fluorescence microscopy (LSFM)	Optical sectioning and high-resolution imaging Imaging depth to 1 cm	Samples must be mounted

Confocal Laser Scanning Microscopy

Confocal laser scanning microscopy (CLSM) have been used widely for high-resolution imaging of biofilm, and in recent years in vivo imaging has become possible [13–17]. This technology is based on a conventional optical microscope but instead of a lamp, a laser beam is focused onto the sample. CLSM offers several advantages over conventional wide-field optical microscopy, including the ability to control depth of field, elimination or reduction of background information away from the focal plane, and the capability to collect serial thin optical sections (0.5–1.5 µm) from thick specimens (ranging up to 50 µm or more) [18]. But CLSM has limitations, such as the limited number of excitation wavelengths available with common lasers which occur over very narrow bands and are expensive to produce [19], limited speed due to point-by-point imaging, the harmful nature of high-intensity laser irradiation to living cells and tissues that can cause photo damage [20], and the high cost of operation [21]. Its effectiveness can be expanded using staining techniques including fluorescence in situ hybridization (FISH), some of which can be used in vivo. For example, FISH techniques combined with CLSM have been used to image natural heterogeneous biofilm on fixed orthodon-tic appliances [22]. Indeed, CLSM has been used in various medical fields including dentistry, oto-rhinolaryngology, and obstetrics [23] to evaluate biofilm, and many attempts including spinning disc confocal laser scanning microscopy have been made to overcome the identified disadvantages [24]. Despite these numerous efforts, natural oral biofilm in the oral cavity has not successfully been imaged using CLSM without staining of some sort to enhance contrast. Typically, oral biofilm studies using CLSM have been performed in vitro or using a variety of biofilm growth media including discs in the oral cavity [25–27]. In vitro oral biofilm models tend to involve limited numbers of species, and they are created under artificial conditions that still cannot adequately reflect the physiological situation in the mouth [28–30].

Two Photon and Multiphoton Microscopy

First described in 1990 by Winfried Denk and James Strickler [31, 32], multiphoton (two or three photon) microscopy was developed to overcome some of the seminal disadvantages of conventional CLSM. This fluorescence imaging technique uses near-infrared excitation light to elicit fluorescence in selective tissue components or materials. It can also excite fluorescent dyes in tissue explants and in tissue or animal models [33]. Multiphoton fluorescence microscopy (MPM) also has been used to image oral biofilm and calculus [34, 35], whose microstructure it reveals very effectively (Figs. 1 and 2). However, similar to CSLM, although to a somewhat lesser degree, above certain intensities MPM can lead to impaired cellular reproduction, formation of giant cells, oxidative stress, and apoptosis-like cell death [36, 37].

Atomic Force Microscopy

Also known as scanning probe microscopy (SPM), atomic force microscopy was introduced by Binnig et al. in 1986 [38]. Using this technol-

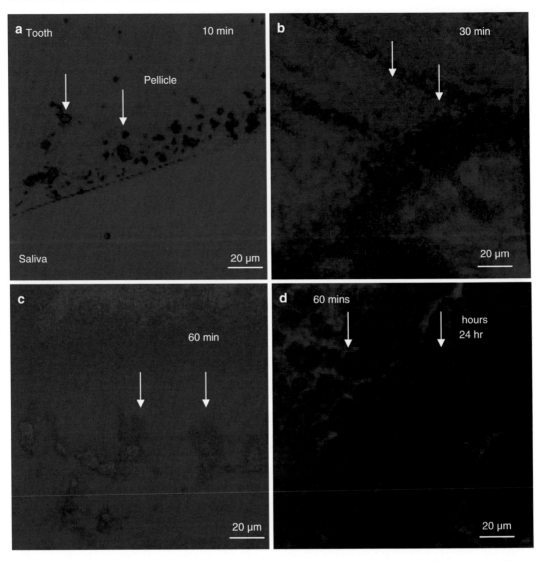

Fig. 1 Progressive growth and development of pellicle (white arrows) on the same tooth sample. Top view of 3D-reconstructed MPM images at progressive saliva incubation time points. (**a**) 10-min incubation. (**b**) 30-min incubation. (**c**) 60-min incubation. Blue signal originates from tooth and saliva, pink and red signals from salivary pellicle. Over time, the number and diameter of pellicle islands gradually increase. (**d**) 24-h incubation. Thick layer of biofilm covers the pellicle. (Figure Courtesy P.W.S)

ogy, researchers were able to establish that the dental pellicle is a stiff, viscoelastic solid with a dense undulating morphology [39]. In addition to providing microstructural information, AFM can also analyze the electronic properties of a sample surface at an atomic resolution level [40]. Using this technology, the nanoscale morphology of bacteria within biofilms can be elucidated [41]. For example, S. mutans *within a biofilm* was characterized at a nanoscale level of resolution [42]. Moreover, associated nano-indentation techniques uniquely permit the detection and characterization of salivary pellicle [43]. While CLSM is useful for identifying specific proteins subsequent to labelling with markers or antibodies, AFM can be used to image unstained macromolecular structures in fixed and living cells [44]. However, because AFM images are obtained by

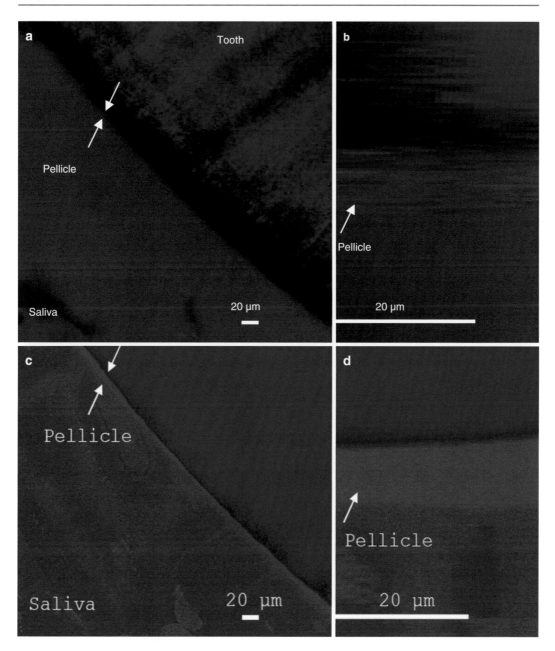

Fig. 2 MPM images showing pellicle growth and development over time (white arrow). (**a**) Tooth incubated in saliva for 30 min. Top view of 3D-reconstructed images. (**b**) Optically sectioned lateral view of (**a**). Coarse layers and voids in the pellicle layer are clearly visible. (**c**) Same tooth incubated in saliva for 120 min. Increased thickness of pellicle layer is visible. (**d**) Inner structure of pellicle layer is more dense and compact than at earlier time point. (Figure Courtesy P.W.S)

measuring forces on a sharp tip that are created by its proximity to the sample surface [38, 45], this technology can only image the cell membrane surfaces of biological samples and cannot directly visualize the interior of the cell [38, 45].

Light Sheet Fluorescence Microscopy

Light sheet fluorescence microscopy (LSFM) also called selective plane illumination microscopy (SPIM) or ultramicroscopy is a fluorescent light microscope imaging technique which is differentiated from CLSM in that it does not require a spatial pinhole to eliminate out of focus light. It was first described by Henry Siedentopf and Richard Adolf Zsigmondy in 1903, who were awarded the Nobel Prize for this work in 1925 [46]. LSFM functions as a combined non-destructive microtome and microscope that uses a plane of light to optically section and view samples with subcellular resolution. This technique is well suited for imaging deep within transparent structures such as biofilm or entire organisms, and because samples are exposed to only a thin plane of light, specimen photobleaching and phototoxicity are minimized compared to wide-field fluorescence, confocal, or multiphoton microscopy. Three-dimensional imaging is possible using LSFM [47]. Compared with confocal and two-photon microscopy, LSFM is able to image samples up to a thickness of 1 cm [37]. Despite its many advantages, LSFM applications to oral biofilm imaging and the oral cavity in general are still lacking, primarily because samples must be mounted prior to imaging. A common method of LSFM sample preparation is sample embedding in an agarose cylinder [47], which is clearly not suitable for biofilm imaging.

Need for New Technology

The greatest disadvantage of many of the aforementioned imaging devices is that they cannot be applied directly in the oral cavity. Biofilm within its oral environment is complex and dynamic. From the moment that it is extracted from the oral cavity, its properties change. Even within the oral biofilm itself, the bacteria are not uniformly distributed. Microcolonies aggregate in various shapes and size. It is for this reason that researchers have turned to techniques such as liquid chromatography-mass spectrometry to analyze

Table 3 The required elements for imaging oral biofilm in situ

Direct application to the oral cavity
No physical or chemical preparation of the biofilm required
None or minimal effects on bacteria and cells
Standardized images available for purposes of quantification and comparison

the proteome of salivary pellicle proteins for mapping bacterial presence and properties [1]. This allows the identification of various organisms such as *Actinomyces naeslundii, Steprococcus oralis, Streptococcus mutans, Fusobacterium nucleatum, Veillonella dispar, Candida albicans* in the salivary pellicle [48]. The bacterial species diversity in the oral cavity indicate is estimated at approximately 500 species [49] (Table 3).

Optical Coherence Tomography

Optical coherence tomography (OCT) is a high-resolution optical technique that permits minimally invasive imaging of near-surface abnormalities in complex tissue. OCT combines principles similar to those of ultrasonic imaging. Whereas ultrasound produces images from back-scattered sound "echoes," OCT uses infrared light waves that reflect off the internal microstructure within the biological tissues. Cross-sectional images of tissues are constructed in real time, at near-histologic resolution. This permits in vivo noninvasive imaging of the macroscopic characteristics of surface and subsurface tissues. Two-dimensional images may be combined to generate 3D images that can be sectional and manipulated in many ways. In vivo OCT images are acquired in seconds or less using a handheld probe; therefore, they can be used in the clinical setting [26]. Higher resolution in vivo OCT imaging is possible by using optical coherence microscopy (OCM) [50, 51].

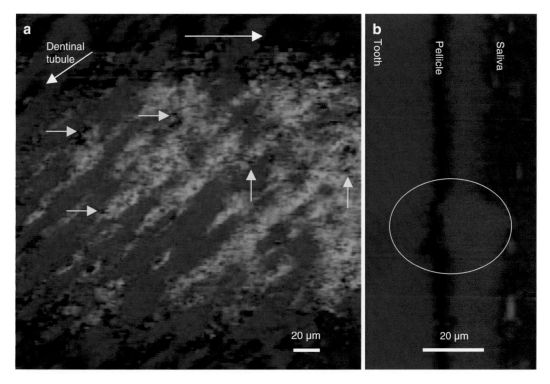

Fig. 3 Low- and high-resolution OCM images using fluorescein stain showing the pellicle after 120-min incubation in saliva. (**a**) Top view of 3D-reconstructed image. The fluorescein is seen as a pink stain at the saliva/tooth interface (arrows). (**b**) Optically sectioned lateral view of 3D-reconstructed image showing pellicle presence and structure in pink. The white circle indicates an area where the attachment between the pellicle and the underlying tooth is evident. (Figure Courtesy P.W.S)

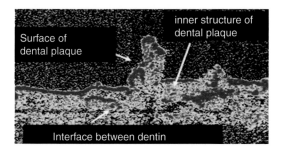

Fig. 4 High-resolution in vivo OCT image showing a vertical optical section of human subgingival dental plaque on the dentin surface of the tooth root. As well as mapping high-resolution image of outer surface of dental plaque, the inner structure, and interface between dentin and dental plaque (the base of plaque) are also distinguishable. (Figure Courtesy J.H.B)

OCT or OCM can be combined with in vivo multiphoton microscopy (MPM), generating high-resolution imaging of specific tissue components and fluorescence using many wavelengths of light [52]. Using combined OCT and OCM, noninvasive imaging of physiological, pathological, and preventive processes becomes possible (Fig. 3). Thus, OCT is well suited for in vivo oral biofilm imaging, overcoming many of the limitations of conventional plaque imaging tools. Figure 4 shows an OCT image of undisturbed dental plaque on an extracted human molar (Fig. 4). The salivary pellicle can also be imaged effectively (Fig. 5).

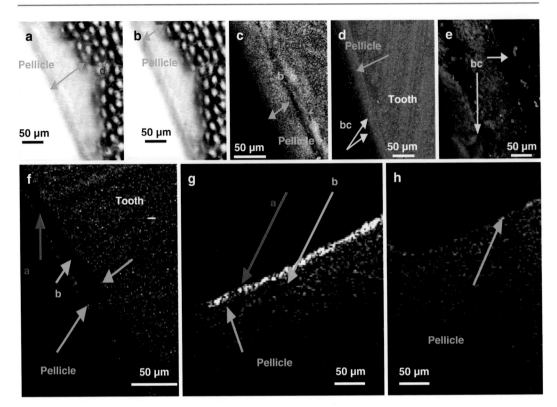

Fig. 5 (**a, b**) OCT images of dentinal surface and the overlying tooth pellicle and cross-sectional images of dentinal tubules (**d**). (**c**) MPM gray scale image showing outer (**a**) and inner (**b**) pellicle layers; (**d, e**) MPM fluorescence images showing pellicle and bacterial clusters (bc); (**f**) MPM gray scale image of tooth after rinsing with a commercial mouth rinse containing 21.6% alcohol. The pellicle remains unchanged. (**g, h**) OCT images before (**g**) and after (**h**) wiping the tooth with 99% isopropyl rubbing alcohol for 1 min. Very little pellicle remains afterwards (**h**). (Figure Courtesy J.H.B)

Practical Considerations

Biofilm formation requires the firm attachment of salivary glycoproteins or salivary pellicle to the tooth surface. This salivary pellicle forms immediately after tooth brushing [53], and it provides the basis for subsequent development of dental plaque. The ability to image oral biofilm is crucial for analyzing the effects of various preventive and interventional approaches to biofilm control [54]. However, quantitative biofilm imaging is challenging due to the complex, heterogeneous, dynamic properties of biofilms [55]. Oral bacteria in plaque do not exist as independent entities but function as a coordinated, spatially organized and fully metabolically integrated microbial community, the properties of which differ considerably from the sum of the component species [56].

Thus, multimodality techniques that combine traditional approaches (such as bioassays) with innovative imaging capabilities can provide the multi-factorial information to map out the complex properties of biofilm structures [57].

Another important factor for ensuring the relevance of intra-oral imaging is image co-localization, or the ability to image consecutively at exactly the same location in the mouth over time. This can be accomplished through various imaging jigs or probe holders tailored to specific site and use (Figs. 6 and 7). Using such devices, biofilm can be quantified at specific time points, locations, or to evaluate specific preventive or interventional approaches relevant to biofilm-related conditions including dental caries, periodontal diseases, and peri-implantitis (Fig. 8). Figure 9 shows the ability of standardized,

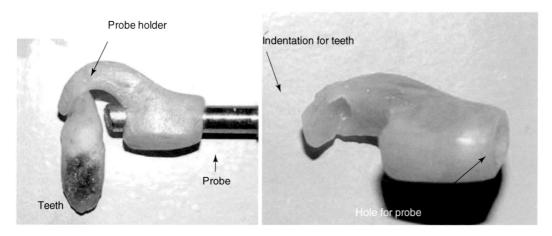

Fig. 6 Prototype intra-oral imaging probe holder. The probe location is accurately controlled by its placement through a slot within the probe body. The custom-fabricated probe body is reproducibly fixated through a custom groove fitting onto an adjacent tooth (Figure Courtesy J.H.B.)

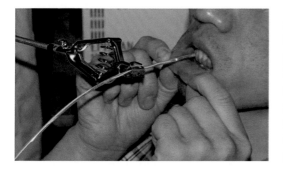

Fig. 7 Prototype extra-oral imaging probe holder. To ensure reproducible re-imaging at exactly the same location during multiple imaging events and to minimize movement artifacts, a multi-joint imaging probe holder for OCT imaging was fabricated. In the future, this multi-joints holder can be replaced with a robotic arm for automatic programmed imaging localization (Figure Courtesy J.H.B.)

co-localized OCM and MPM imaging techniques to map and quantify the effects of various anti-plaque agents [58, 59]. In vivo imaging resolution and selectivity can be further enhanced by the use of advanced dyes and nanoparticles. A preliminary study demonstrated the successful use of 15 nm and 18 nm diameter gold nanoparticles to visualize early pellicle development after tooth cleaning (Fig. 10).

Fig. 8 In vivo, in situ OCT images of human dental calculus on the lingual surface of the lower anterior incisors. (**a–c**) 3D-reconstructed OCT images. (**d**) 2 D raw image prepared by optical sectioning of a 3D image (Figure Courtesy J.H.B.)

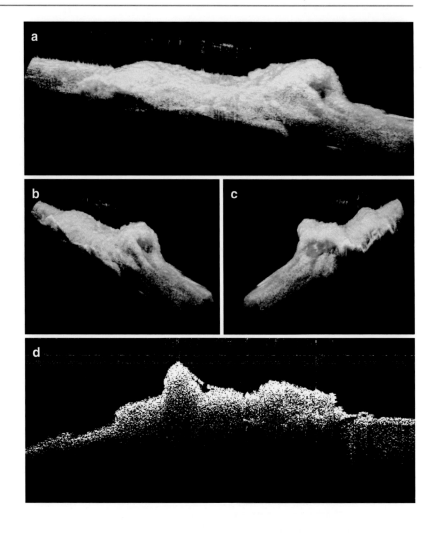

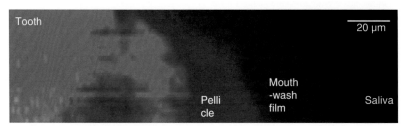

Fig. 9 Lateral 3D OCM image with superimposed MPM image of a tooth after rinsing with mouthwash (Listerine®). The tooth surface (green), overlying pellicle (red), film of mouthwash (purple), and saliva ((dark) brown) are all visible (Figure Courtesy J.H.B.)

Fig. 10 Multimodality images showing use of gold nanoparticles for imaging the salivary pellicle. An extracted tooth was incubated in saliva mixed with 15 nm diameter gold nanoparticles and fluorescein for 120 min. (**a**) OCM image; (**b**) MPM image; (**c**) Combined OCM and MPM image. Zone a; Saliva. Gold nanoparticle (arrow) and fluorescein are present in this zone. Zone b; Pellicle. Fewer gold nanoparticles and strong fluorescein signal (arrow) are visible. Zone c; Outer dentin surface. Gold nanoparticles are unable to penetrate, but there is a strong fluorescein signal that permits visual differentiation between saliva, pellicle, and dentin (Figure Courtesy J.H.B.)

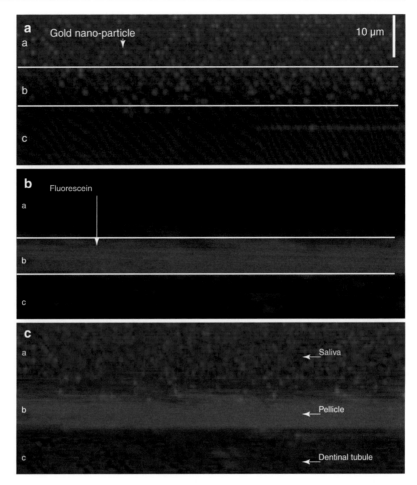

Conclusion

Mapping and quantifying oral biofilm in its natural environment remains challenging. Recent advances in imaging technologies such as OCT and MPM including multiple reference optical coherence tomography (MR-OCT) [59] are rapidly expanding our abilities to characterize and monitor oral biofilm within its natural environment. Applying cutting edge artificial intelligence machine learning techniques to such imaging data will enhance its value and relevance to improving oral health and understanding the complex role that oral biofilm plays in it.

References

1. Whittaker C, Ridgway H, Olson BH. Evaluation of cleaning strategies for removal of biofilms from reverse-osmosis membranes. Appl Environ Microbiol. 1984;48(2):395–403.
2. Chandki R, Banthia P, Banthia R. Biofilms: a microbial home. J Indian Soc Periodontol. 2011;15(2):111–4. https://doi.org/10.4103/0972-124X.84377.
3. Hannig M, Fiebiger M, Güntzer M, Döbert A, Zimehl R, Nekrasheych Y. Protective effect of the in situ formed short-term salivary pellicle. Arch Oral Biol. 2004;49:903–10.
4. Nieuw Amerongen AV, Oderkerk CH, Driessen AA. Role of mucins from human whole saliva in the protection of tooth enamel against demineralization in vitro. Caries Res. 1987;21:297–309.
5. Hannig C, Wasser M, Becker K, Hannig M, Huber K, Attin T. Influence of different restorative materials on

lysozyme and amylase activity of the salivary pellicle in situ. J Biomed Mater Res Part A. 2006;78A:755–61.

6. Zahradnik RT, Moreno EC, Burke EJ. Effect of salivary pellicle on enamel subsurface demineralization in vitro. J Dent Res. 1976;55:664–70.

7. Hannig M, Hess NJ, Hoth-Hannig W, de Vrese M. Influence of salivary pellicle formation time on enamel demineralization-an *in situ* pilot study. Clin Oral Investig. 2003;7:158–61.

8. Roberts AP, Mullany P. Oral biofilms: a reservoir of transferable, bacterial, antimicrobial resistance. Expert Rev Anti Infect Ther. 2010;8(12):1441–50.

9. Ahimou F, Semmens MJ, Novak PJ, Haugstad G. Biofilm cohesiveness measurement using a novel atomic force microscopy methodology. Appl Environ Microbiol. 2007;73(9):2897–904.

10. Schilling KM, Bowe WH. Glucans synthesized in situ in experimental salivary pellicle function as specific binding sites for streptococcus mutans. Infect Immun. 1992;60:284–95.

11. Gong K, Mailloux L, Herzberg MC. Salivary film express a complex, macromolecular binding site for streptococcus sanguis. J Biol Chem. 2000;275:8970–4.

12. Dobell C. Antony Van Leewenhoek and his 'little animals'. The first observations on entozoic protozoa and bacteria. New York: Russell and Russell, Inc.; 1958. p. 236–56.

13. Karygianni L, Follo M, Hellwig E, Burghardt D, Wolkewitz M, Anderson A, et al. Microscope-based imaging platform for large-scale analysis of oral biofilms. Appl Environ Microbiol. 2012;78(24):8703–11.

14. Zaura-Arite E, van Marle J, ten Cate JM. Conforcal microscopy study of undisturbed and chlorhexidine-treated dental biofilm. J Dent Res. 2016;80(5):1436–40.

15. Wood SR, Kirkham J, Marsh PD, Shore RC, Nattress B, Robinson C. Architecture of intact natural human plaque biofilms studied by confocal laser scanning microscopy. J Dent Res. 2016;79(1):21–7.

16. Dige I, Nilsson H, Kilian M, Nyvad B. *In situ* identification of streptococci and other bacteria in initial dental biofilm by confocal laser scanning microscopy and fluorescence *in situ* hybridization. Eur J Oral Sci. 2007;115(6):459–67.

17. Netuschil L, Reich E, Unteregger G, Schulean A, Brecx M. A pilot study of confocal laser scanning microcopy for the assessment of undisturbed dental plaque vitality and topography. Arch Oral Biol. 1998;43(4):277–85.

18. Sandison D, Webb W. Background rejection and signal-to-noise optimization in the confocal and alternative fluorescence microscopes. Appl Opt. 1994;33:603–10.

19. Gratton E, van de Ven MJ. Laser sources for confocal microscopy. In: Pawley JB, editor. Handbook of biological confocal microscopy. New York: Plenum Press; 1995. p. 69–98.

20. Ashkin A, Dziedzic JM, Yamane T. Optical trapping and manipulation of single cells using infrared laser beams. Nature. 1987;330:769–71.

21. Claxton NS, Fellers TJ, Davidson MW. Laser scanning confocal microscopy. Tallahassee: Department of Optical Microscopy and Digital Imaging, Florida State University; 2006. http://www.olympusconfocal.com/theory/LSCMIntro.pdf.

22. Klug B, Rodler C, Koller M, Wimmer G, Kessler H, Grube M, et al. Oral biofilm analysis of palatal expanders by fluorescence in-situ hybridization and confocal laser scanning microscopy. J Vis Exp. 2011;56:2967.

23. Gabriela PM. Confocal scanning laser microscopy in the study of biofilm formation in tissues of the upper airway in otolaryngologic disease. Miscosc Sci Technol Appl Educ. 2010;3:590–6.

24. Nakano A. Spinning disk confocal microscopy—a cutting-edge tool for imaging of membrane traffic. Cell Struct Funct. 2002;27(5):349–55.

25. Tomas I, Henderson B, Biz P, Donos N. In vivo oral biofilm analysis by conforcal laser scanning microscopy: methodological approaches. Miscosco Sci Technol Appl Educ. 2010;3:597–606.

26. Baek JH, Krasieva T, Tang S, Ahn Y, Kim C, Vu D, Chen Z, Wilder-Smith P. Optical approach to the salivary pellicle. J Biomed Opt. 2009;14(4):044001.

27. Wood SR, Kirkham J, Marsh PD, Shore RC, Nattress B, Robinson C. Architecture of intact natural human plaque biofilms studied by confocal laser scanning microscopy. J Dent Res. 2000;79:21–7.

28. Wecke J, Kersten T, Madela K, Moter A, Göbel UB, Friedmann A, Bernimoulin J. A novel technique for monitoring the development of bacterial biofilms in human periodontal pockets. FEMS Microbiol Lett. 2000;191:95–101.

29. Auschill TM, Hellwig E, Sculean A, Hein N, Arweiller NB. Impact of the intraoral location on the rate of biofilm growth. Clin Oral Investig. 2004;8:97–101.

30. Watson PS, Pontefract HA, Devine DA, Shore RC, Nattres BR, Kirkham J, Robinson C. Penetration of fluoride into natural plaque biofilms. J Dent Res. 2005;84:451–5.

31. Neu TR, Kuhlicke U, Lawrence JR. Assessment of fluorochromes for two-photon laser scanning microscopy of biofilms. Appl Environ Microbiol. 2002;68(2):901–9.

32. Denk W, Strickler JH, Webb WW. Two-photon laser scanning fluorescence microscopy. Science. 248:73–6.

33. Zipfel WR, Williams RM, Webb WW. Nonlinear magic: multiphoton microscopy in the biosciences. Nat Biotechnol. 2003;21:1369–77.

34. Maeda K, Tribble GD, Tucker CM, Anaya C, Shizukuishi S, Lewis JP, Demuth DR, Lamont RJ. A porphyromonas gingivalis tyrosine phosphatase is a multifunctional regulator of virulence attributes. Mol Microbiol. 2008;69(5):1153–64.

35. Tung OH, Lee SY, Lai YL, Chen HF. Characteristics of subgingival calculus detection by multiphoton fluorescence microscopy. J Biomed Opt. 2011;16(6):066017.

36. König K. Multiphoton microscopy in life sciences. J Microsc. 2000;200(2):83–104.

37. Bode J, Kruwel T, Tews B. Light sheet fluorescence microscopy combined with optical clearing methods as a novel imaging tool in biomedical research. Eur Med J. 2017;1:67–74.

38. Binnig G, Quate CF, Gerber C. Atomic force microscope. Phys Rev Lett. 1986;56:930–3.

39. Dickinson ME, Mann AB. Nanomechanics and morphology of salivary pellicle. J Mater Res. 2006;21(8):1996–2002.

40. Howland R, Benatar L, Park scientific instruments. A practical guide to scanning probe microscopy. Park scientific instruments; 1996.

41. Germano F, Bramanti E, Arcuri C, Cecchetti F, Cicciu M. Atomic force microcopy of bacteria from periodontal subgingival biofilm: preliminary study results. Eur J Dent. 2013;7(2):152–8.

42. Sharma S, Lavender S, Guo L, Gimzewski JK. Nasoscale characterization of effect of L-arginine on S. mutans biofilm adhesion by atomic force microscopy. Microbiology. 2014;160:1466–73.

43. Dickinson ME, Mann AB. Nanoscale characterisation of salivary pellicle. MRS Proc. 844. https://doi.org/10.1557/PROC-844-Y2.3/R2.3.

44. Meller K, Theiss C. Atomic force microscopy and confocal laser scanning microscopy on the cytoskeleton of permeabilized and embedded cells. Ultramicroscopy. 2005;106:320–5.

45. Kumar S, Hoh JH. Probing the machinery of intracelluer trafficking with the atomic force microscope. Traffic. 2001;2(11):746–56.

46. Siedentopf H. Visualization and size measurement of ultramicroscopic particles, with special application to gold-colored ruby glass. Ann Phys. 1903;10:1–39.

47. Santi PA. Light sheet fluorescence microscopy. J Histochem Cytochem. 2011;59(2):129–38.

48. Cavalcanti IM, Ricomini FAP, Lucena-Ferreira SC, da Silva WJ, Paes Leme AF, Senna PM, Del Bel Cury AA. Salivary pellicle composition and multispecies biofilm developed on titanium nitrided by cold plasma. Arch Oral Biol. 2014;59(7):695–7.

49. Kolenbrander PE, Anderson RN, Palmar RJ Jr, et al. Communication among oral bacteria. Microbiol Mol Biol Rev. 2002;66(3):486–505.

50. Vokes DE, Jackson R, Guo S, Perez A, Su J, Ridgway M, Armstrong WB, Chen Z, Wong BJ. Optical coherence tomography-enhanced microlaryngoscopy: preliminary report of a noncontact optical coherence tomography system integrated with a surgical microscope. Ann Otol Rhinol Laryngol. 2008;117(7):538–47.

51. Chelliyil RG, Ralston TS, Marks DL, Boppart SA. High speed processing architecture for spectral-domain optical coherence microscopy. J Biomed Opt. 2008;13(4):44013.

52. Sumen C, Mempel TR, Mazo IB, von Andrian UH. Intravital microscopy: visualizing immunity in context. Immunity. 2004;21(3):315–29.

53. Huang R, Li M, Gregory RL. Bacterial interactions in dental biofilm. Virulence. 2011;2:435–44.

54. Corbin A, Pitts B, Parker A, Stewart PS. Antimicrobial penetration and efficancy in an in vitro oral biofilm model. Antimicrob Agents Chemother. 2011;55(7):3338–44.

55. Baker PJ, Pintar AL, Lin-Gibson S, Lin NJ, Lopez-Perez D. Evaluating the activity of an anti-biofilm agent via imaging. *BioImaging Informatics Conference*. 2015.

56. March PD. Dental plaque as a microbial biofilm. Caries Res. 2004;38(3):204–11.

57. Ajdaharian J, Dadkhah M, Sabokpey S, Biren-Fetz J, Chung NE, Wink C, Wilder-Smith P. Multimodality imaging of the effects of a novel dentifrice on oral biofilm. Lasers Surg Med. 2014;46(7):546–52.

58. Quintas V, Prada-López I, Prados-Frutos JC, Tomás I. In situ antimicrobial activity on oral biofilm: essential oils vs. 0.2% chlorhexidine. Clin Oral Investig. 2015;19(1):97–107.

59. McNamara PM, Dsouza R, O'Riordan C, Collins S, O'Brien P, Wilson C, Hogan J, Leahy MJ. Development of a first-generation miniature multiple reference optical coherence tomography imaging device. J Biomed Opt. 2016;21(12):126020.

Oral Cancer

Diana Messadi, Anh D. Le, Takako Tanaka,
and Petra Wilder-Smith

Abstract

Because the clinical appearance of oral mucosal lesions is not an adequate indicator of their diagnosis, status or risk level, additional means of assessing these lesions are needed to ensure accurate and early detection, diagnosis, treatment planning, and execution, as well as monitoring. Early diagnosis is the most important determinant of oral cancer outcomes, yet the majority of oral cancers are detected late, when outcomes are poor. This chapter addresses emerging optical imaging modalities for evaluating oral soft tissue conditions such as dysplasia and malignancy. Desirable attributes include: providing clinical decision-making guidance to improve outcomes, ease and speed of use, appropriate cost for the indicated setting, safety (absence of ionizing radiation), patient-friendly probes, and reliability. In this chapter, the principles behind optical diagnostic approaches, their feasibility and applicability for imaging oral tissues, and their potential usefulness as a tool in the diagnosis of oral cancer and potentially premalignant lesions are reviewed.

D. Messadi
Section of Oral Medicine, Division of Oral Biology & Medicine, UCLA School of Dentistry, Los Angeles, CA, USA

A. D. Le
Department of Oral and Maxillofacial Surgery, University of Pennsylvania School of Dental Medicine, Philadelphia, PA, USA

T. Tanaka
University of Pennsylvania School of Dental Medicine, Philadelphia, PA, USA

P. Wilder-Smith (✉)
Beckman Laser Institute and Medical Clinic, University of California, Irvine, CA, USA
e-mail: pwsmith@uci.edu

Background

Worldwide, 650,000 incident cases and 223,000 deaths from oral and oropharyngeal cancer (OC) are reported each year [1, 2]. In the USA, 54,000 OC cases and 13,500 deaths occur annually [3]. HPV-associated OCs are increasing at an alarming rate, and up to 70% of oropharyngeal cancers are HPV-associated [4] (Table 1).

The mean 5-year survival rate in the USA for OC approximates 50% and has not improved over decades despite significant advances in treatment [3]. Additionally, 1–10% of the US population manifests oral potentially premalignant lesions (OPMLs) [5, 6] with a risk of malignant transformation of up to 35% [7–9]. The poor survival rate for OC is mainly due to late diagnosis [10], as the largest single variable affecting survival is the cancer's stage at diagnosis [3, 11–14]. Since more than two-thirds of OC lesions are detected late, treatment outcomes and prognoses are poor [3, 15].

Oral carcinogenesis is typically a multi-step process wherein the mucosa progresses through a

Table 1 Overview of chapter content: techniques for oral diagnosis

Existing techniques	Available minimally invasive methods	New imaging methods	View into the future
Clinical examination Risk assessment Toluidine blue stain Surgical biopsy Histopathology	Autofluorescence Chemiluminescence	Optical coherence tomography Smartphone-based autofluorescence	High-resolution fiberoptic microendoscopy

series of OPMLs before becoming invasive OC. OPMLs require regular monitoring to identify any increase in OC risk because of our inability to predict malignant change in individuals [16]. Yet compliance with monitoring is typically poor [17]. Thus, there clearly exists an urgent and widespread unmet need for alternate approaches to surveillance in persons with OPMLs [3, 15].

Survival and quality of life of high-risk individuals are dependent on our ability to detect and monitor early-stage OCs and OPMLs. The 5-year survival rate for those with localized OC at diagnosis approximates 80% [14]. It drops to 20% if cancer has spread at diagnosis [14]. Marginalized at-risk populations commonly lack access to health care and have low health literacy, as well as poor adherence to referral and follow-up, so that they carry an increased risk of late detection and treatment leading to poor outcomes [18–20].

A wide range of assistive imaging-based approaches to detecting and diagnosing oral potential premalignancy and malignancy are under investigation. Some of these have been available for many years, and there is a considerable amount of information available with regard to their strengths and weaknesses. Others are very new, and their effectiveness is still under investigation. For the purposes of organization, this chapter has been divided into the following topic groupings: Fluorescence and Spectroscopy, Induced Fluorescence, Chemiluminescence, Optical Coherence Tomography, and View to the Future.

Fluorescence and Spectroscopy

A number of methods based on the principles of tissue fluorescence have been described for use in the oral cavity, including exogenous fluores-cence, autofluorescence spectroscopy, and autofluorescence imaging.

Tissue autofluorescence has been applied for screening and diagnosis of pre-cancer and early cancer of the lung, uterine cervix, skin and, more recently, of the oral cavity. It is a phenomenon whereby an extrinsic light source is used to excite endogenous fluorophores such as certain amino acids, metabolic products, and structural proteins. Spectroscopy or autofluorescence imaging can provide information about these altered light interaction properties.

During the disease process, the altered cellular structure (e.g., hyperkeratosis, hyperchromatin, and increased cellular/nuclear pleomorphism) and/or metabolism affect tissue interaction with light. Within the oral mucosa, the most relevant fluorophores are nicotinamide adenine dinucleotide (NADH) and flavin adenine dinucleotide (FAD) in the epithelium, and collagen cross-links in the stroma. These fluorophores absorb photons from the exogenous light source, resulting in the emission of lower energy photons which present clinically as fluorescence [21]. Each fluorophore is associated with specific excitation and emission wavelengths. Irradiation of healthy oral mucosa at wavelengths between 375 and 440 nm elicits a pale green autofluorescence when viewed through a selective, narrowband filter. Proper light filtration is crucial to exclude the intense excitation light and permit visualization of the considerably less intense and narrow autofluorescence signal. Dysplastic and malignant oral tissues produce a considerably weaker green autofluorescence signal due to fluorophore disruption, resulting in a darker appearance compared to the surrounding healthy tissue [22] (Fig. 1).

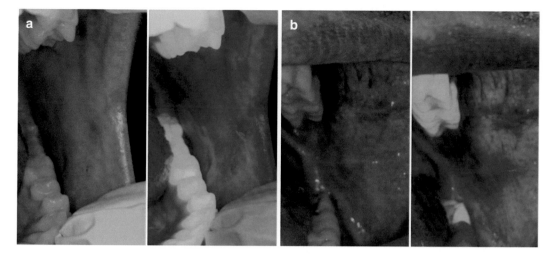

Fig. 1 (**a**, **b**) Clinical (LHS) and autofluorescence (RHS) images of healthy (**a**) and dysplastic (**b**) mucosa. The healthy mucosa shows a strong, uniform green autofluorescence signal, whereas areas of dysplasia appear dark. (Courtesy P.W.S.)

In the last decade, several forms of autofluorescence technology have been developed for inspection of the oral mucosa.

The VELscope™ System

VELscope™ utilizes blue light excitation between 400 and 460 nm wavelength to enhance visibility of oral mucosal abnormalities by direct tissue autofluorescence. At these excitation wavelengths, normal oral mucosa is associated with a pale green fluorescence when viewed through a filter, whereas abnormal tissue is associated with a loss of autofluorescence and appears dark. Neoplastic tissues are expected to cause fluorescent visualization loss and thus appear as a dark area [23]. A wide range of studies have investigated the effectiveness of the VELscope™ system as an adjunct to visual examination in the detection of OSCC and OPMD. These studies were mainly cross-sectional and were carried out in clinics of countries such as the UK [24], Canada [25], Germany [26–28], Italy [21], the USA [29, 30], Poland [31], and India [32]. These clinical studies demonstrated sensitivities for detecting malignancy and OPMD ranging from 22 to 100%, and specificities ranging from 16 to 100%. Most studies concluded that VELscope™ can be useful in aiding detection of oral precursor malignant lesions [28, 30, 33]. Using histology as the comparative gold standard, VELscope™ demonstrated high sensitivity and specificity in identifying areas of dysplasia and malignancy that extended beyond the clinically evident tumors [23, 34–37].

Several studies have additionally investigated the effectiveness of the VELscope™ system as an adjunct to visual examination for (1) improving the distinction between normal and abnormal tissues (both benign and malignant changes), (2) differentiating between benign and dysplastic/malignant changes, and (3) identifying dysplastic/malignant lesions that are visible to the naked eye under white light. Whether it can distinguish between dysplasia and benign inflammatory lesions is questioned. Benign inflammatory conditions can result in an increased blood supply to a lesion. The increased hemoglobin content (chromophores) may absorb light and cause fluorescence visualization loss mimicking neoplasia [29, 30].

Clinical Usage [38]

Prior to utilizing the VELscope™ system, clinicians should conduct a thorough extra-oral and intra-oral examination both visually and manually, palpating all the structures of the head and neck. Then, the intra-oral examination should be repeated by viewing the oral cavity through the VELscope™ handpiece while maintaining a distance of approximately 5 cm from the oral tissues to optimize autofluorescence visualization (Fig. 2).

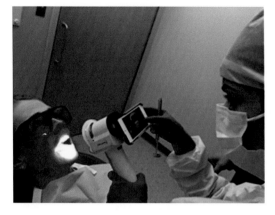

Fig. 2 VELscope system in use. (Courtesy T.T.)

Abnormal tissue will typically appears as an irregular, dark area that stands out against the green fluorescence pattern of the surrounding healthy tissue. Any area with a suspicious appearance should be reevaluated under white light to identify what might have caused the region to appear abnormal. Indicators of heightened risk may include: a strong loss of fluorescence signal, reduced autofluorescence in a high-risk location (e.g., lateral/ventral tongue), unilateral, asymmetrical, or irregular shaped presentation, as well as lesion extension over more than one kind of oral structure. Confounding factors may include the following: Inflammation typically appears darker, and this is commonly seen in the buccal mucosa, lateral surfaces of the tongue and hard palate; hyperkeratosis may appear bright.

The Identafi™ System

This device combines autofluorescence and reflectance imaging to provide enhanced visibility of mucosal pathologies such as oral cancer or premalignant dysplasia, as well as microstructural and vascular changes that may not be apparent to the naked eye. The Identafi™ is multi-spectral with three excitation wavelengths, white, 405 nm violet, and green-amber, with the goal of combining multiple optical markers to enhance the clinician's ability to characterize lesion presence, morphology, and vasculature. Studies indicate abnormal tissue has a diffuse vasculature, whereas normal tissue's vasculature is more clearly defined [39]. Visually differentiating between normal and abnormal vasculature

may aid with selecting biopsy sites and margins. Advantages of this device include its lightness, portability, robustness, and simplicity of operation, as well as its easy accessibility to all areas of the oral cavity. In one study researchers demonstrated a sensitivity of 82% and a specificity of 87% in differentiating between neoplastic and non-neoplastic oral conditions [40]. Another study reported sensitivity and specificity of 100% and 91%, respectively, for discriminating between dysplasia and malignancy [41]. Finally, Roblyer et al. [42] reported 96–100% sensitivity and 91–96% specificity for differentiating between normal oral mucosa and dysplasia or malignancy. Results appear to vary between sampling depths, and keratinized vs. non-keratinized tissues [43]. Further investigations are needed to evaluate the clinical utility and effect on OC outcomes of this device.

Clinical Usage

The Identafi™ is a battery operated, handheld multi-spectral oral examination light. Accessories include filtered eyewear and disposable mirrors. Prior to utilizing the system, clinicians should conduct a thorough extra-oral and intra-oral examination both visually and manually, palpating all the structures of the head and neck. Then, the intra-oral examination should be repeated by viewing the oral cavity with the Identafi™ handpiece and disposable dental mirror (Fig. 3). The

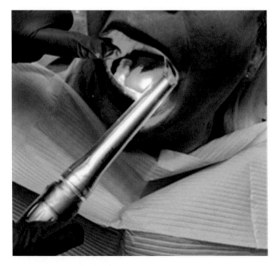

Fig. 3 Indentafi system in use. (Courtesy T.T.)

clinician wears rose colored glasses to examine the oral cavity under all three lights. These glasses filter out the strong excitation light so that tissue autofluorescence and reflectance can be visualized well. Strong white light is used for the initial exam to facilitate detection of any surface changes in the mucosa. Under white light, a lesion may appear raised or thickened and either white or red. Next, the violet light is activated. Dysplastic and malignant tissues appear darker than healthy mucosa because of their loss of fluorescence. Finally, the selector is switched to green-amber light, which enhances normal tissue's reflectance properties so the clinician may more clearly observe lesion margins and the difference between normal and abnormal tissue's vasculature. The green-amber light enhances optical contrast between vasculature and surrounding tissue facilitating visual differentiation between normal and abnormal vasculature. Confounding factors may include fluorescence from certain microorganisms, mold and fungi as well as inflammation.

The Microlux/DL° System

This device consists of a reusable, battery-powered light-emitting diode (LED) light source that provides a blue-white (440 nm range) illumination as an aid to improve the visualization of oral lesions. Light scattering is primarily caused by cell nuclei and organelles in the epithelium and stroma, as well as collagen fibers and cross-links in stroma. Neoplastic tissues exhibit significant changes in their physiological and morphological characteristics that can affect light scattering. During dysplasia and carcinogenesis, epithelial scattering has been shown to increase due to increased nuclear size, increased DNA content, and hyperchromasia [24, 43–45]. Moreover, after rinsing with a 1% acetic acid solution, wide angle side scattering from both the nucleus and the cytoplasm increases [46]. Nuclear protein precipitation is considered to be one of the primary causes of acetowhitening. After rinsing with a mild acetic acid solution, abnormal squamous epithelium appears distinctly white (acetowhite) when viewed under diffuse blue-white light such as that from the *Microlux/DL®* light guide.

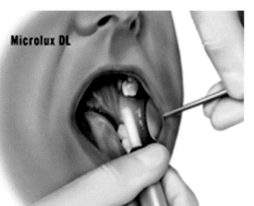

Fig. 4 Microlux system in use. (Courtesy Microlux; permission obtained by T.T.)

Clinical Usage

Clinicians should first conduct a thorough extra-oral and intra-oral examination both visually and manually, palpating all the structures of the head and neck. Next, the patient should rinse with 1% acetic acid solution. After lowering the room light, the Microlux DL tip is placed in the mouth, and the oral cavity inspected with a conventional dental probe to identify any acetowhitened or leukoplakic lesions (Fig. 4).

Chemiluminescence

It was almost 1000 years ago that natural luminescence in living organisms was first reported in Chinese literature, the best-known examples being emission of light from fireflies and glow-worms. The German physician, Henning Brand, discovered phosphorus in 1669, and he based his first report of artificial luminescence (chemiluminescence) on this discovery. Such light emission is the result of relaxation of an excited molecule back to its ground state. The various types of luminescence differ in the source of energy to obtain the excited state: in chemiluminescence, the energy is produced by a chemical reaction which results in the emission of light in a wide range of colors, degrees of intensity and duration [47].

Chemiluminescence has been employed in the field of obstetrics and gynecology for many years as an adjunct for the early detection of cervical cancer and pre-cancer. The technique involves inspection of the cervix following the application of 5% acetic acid with chemiluminescent light. This technique has been translated to oral oncology for the detection of oral pre-cancer and cancer.

The ViziLite® and ViziLite Plus® Systems

Both systems use a disposable chemiluminescent light packet to provide blue-white (440 nm range) illumination within the oral cavity. Under the blue-white illumination, abnormal squamous epithelium is reported to appear distinctly white (acetowhite). The ViziLite Plus® system additionally provides a toluidine blue solution which is intended to mark an acetowhite lesion for subsequent biopsy.

Numerous studies with a wide range of outcomes have investigated the efficacy of ViziLite® in oral pre-cancer and cancer detection [32, 48–58]. Several studies concluded that a chemiluminescent exam using ViziLite® helps to enhance the evaluation of lesion texture and size in comparison with regular incandescent light [53, 59–61]. Indeed, ViziLite® is generally considered to be effective in detecting lesions that are not seen by standard visual examination [32, 49, 55–58]. However, a few studies have reported that no additional lesions were detected or diagnoses made during the use of ViziLite® [50, 52, 55–57]. Several investigators report high diagnostic sensitivity (100%) but low specificity (0–14%) and PPV (18–80%) vs. the gold standard, histopathological diagnosis.

Clinical Usage

The ViziLite® and ViziLite Plus® kits are both single use products that include a light-emitting capsule, a 1% acetic acid solution, and a retractor. The ViziLite Plus® kit additionally contains 1% tolonium chloride for marking acetowhite lesions and a decolorizing rinse. The light-emitting capsule is activated when it is flexed, causing the inner fragile glass vial to break so that the chemicals in the outer and inner compartments react to produce bluish-white light a wavelength of 430–580 nm. The light lasts for approximately 10 min. After a thorough extra-

oral and intra-oral examination, the 1% acetic acid solution is applied, room lights are dimmed and the oral cavity re-inspected using the chemiluminescent stick for illumination. While normal epithelium appears blue, the altered epithelium appears acetowhite. If the ViziLite Plus® kit is being used, the subject then rinses the mouth with 10 mL of 1% tolonium choride and expectorates after 1 min followed by a 20 s rinse with 10 mL of 1% acetic acid before final expectoration. The tolonium chloride produces a deep blue color that aids in the easy visualization and delineation of the chemiluminescent positive area.

Photosensitizers

This technique encompasses the use of external fluorophores such as porphyrins or their precursors to achieve selective localization and fluorescence in areas of pathology [59, 60]. Photosensitizers can be administered topically or systemically. After a delay that permits the fluorophore to reach an adequate concentration in the area of interest, the selective fluorescence in the diseased tissues is imaged and quantified (Fig. 5). Both the timing and the intensity of the photosensitizer-induced fluorescence inform on the level of pathology within a lesion (Fig. 5). Many photosensitizing agents have been studied; however, FDA approval for photosensitizing drugs remains limited. Some promising agents for photodetection include aminolevulinic acid (ALA) (Levulan®), hexyl aminolevulinate (Hexvix®), methyl aminolevulinate (MetvixR), tetra(meta-hydroxyphenyl)chlorin (mTHPC®), as well as porfimer sodium (Photofrin®) [61–65]. In a blinded clinical study of 20 patients with oral neoplasms, diagnostic sensitivity using unaided visual fluorescence diagnosis or fluorescence microscopy approximated 93%. Diagnostic specificity was 95% for visual diagnosis with the naked eye, improving to 97% using fluorescence microscopy [62]. Depending on the photosensitizer and its mode of application (systemic vs. topical), limitations include systemic photosensitization over prolonged periods of time, penetration-related issues, the need

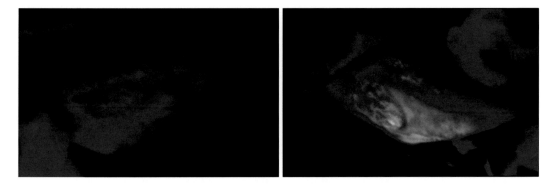

Fig. 5 LHS: Dysplastic lesion of the tongue showing weak red fluorescence 3 h after topical application of the photosensitizer precursor 5-aminolevulinic acid RHS: Squamous cell carcinoma of the tongue showing strong, extensive multi-local red fluorescence 3 h after topical application of the photosensitizer precursor 5-aminolevulinic acid. (Courtesy P.W.S.)

for specialized fluorescence detection and mapping equipment, and lack of specificity when inflammation or scar tissues are present. A recent study using epidermal targeted fluorescent agents by topical applications to oral mucosal lesions combined with in vivo imaging showed encouraging results with regard to lesion detection, margin delineation, and as an adjunct guiding tool for biopsy [66].

Due to practical considerations, and because photosensitizers are generally not FDA-cleared for oral diagnosis, photodynamic detection is unlikely to be applied as a screening aid in dental practice in the USA despite the considerable promise shown by this approach.

Optical Coherence Tomography

Optical coherence tomography (OCT) was first introduced as an imaging technique in biological systems in 1991 [67]. The noninvasive nature of this imaging modality coupled with (1) a penetration depth of 1–3 mm, (2) high-resolution (1–15 μm), real-time image viewing, and (3) capability for cross-sectional as well as 3-D tomographic images, provide excellent prerequisites for in vivo oral screening and diagnosis.

OCT has most often been compared to ultrasound imaging. Both technologies employ backscattered signals reflected from different layers within the tissue to reconstruct structural images, with the latter measuring sound rather than light. The resulting OCT image is a two-dimensional representation of the optical reflection within a tissue sample. Cross-sectional images of tissues are constructed in real time, at near-histologic resolution (approximately 1–15 μm with current technology). These images can be stacked to generate 3-D reconstructions of the target tissue. This permits in vivo noninvasive imaging of epithelial and subepithelial structures, including: (1) depth and thickness, (2) histopathological appearance, and (3) peripheral margins of the lesions. Contrast in OCT images is primarily attributed to differences in light absorption and scattering by the tissues.

Several OCT systems have received FDA approval for clinical use, and OCT is deemed by many as an essential imaging modality in ophthalmology. In vivo image acquisition is facilitated through the use of a flexible fiberoptic OCT probe. The probe is simply placed on the surface of the tissue to generate real-time, immediate surface and sub-surface images of tissue microanatomy and cellular structure, while avoiding the discomfort, delay, and expense of biopsies (Fig. 6).

Several studies have sought to investigate the diagnostic utility of in vivo OCT to detect and diagnose oral premalignancy and malignancy [68, 69]. In a blinded study involving 50 patients with suspicious lesions including oral leukoplakia or erythroplakia, the effectiveness of OCT was evaluated for detecting oral dysplasia and malignancy [69]. OCT images of dysplastic lesions revealed visible epithelial thickening, loss of epithelial stratification, and epithelial downgrowth (Fig. 7). Areas of oral squamous cell carcinoma of the buccal mucosa were identified in the OCT images by the absence or disruption of the basement membrane, an epithelial layer that was highly variable in thickness, with areas of erosion and extensive epithelial down-growth and invasion into the subepithelial layers (Fig. 7). Statistical analysis of the data gathered in this study substantiated the ability of in vivo OCT to detect and diagnose oral premalignancy and malignancy in the oral cavity, with excellent diagnostic accuracy. For detecting carcinoma in situ or squamous cell carcinoma (SCC) vs. noncancer, sensitivity and specificity were both 93%; for detecting SCC vs. all other pathologies, sensitivity was 93% and specificity 97%.

In another study of 97 patients using OCT imaging to detect neoplasia in the oral cavity

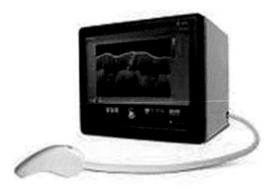

Fig. 6 OCT system. (Courtesy Santec; permission obtained P.W.S.)

[70], the results revealed that the main diagnostic criterion for high-grade dysplasia/carcinoma in situ was the lack of a layered structural pattern. Diagnosis based on this criterion for dysplastic/malignant versus benign/reactive conditions achieved a sensitivity of 83% and specificity of 98% with an inter-observer agreement value of 0.76. This study concluded that OCT, with high sensitivity and specificity combined with good inter-observer agreement, is a promising imaging modality for noninvasive evaluation of tissue sites suspicious for high-grade dysplasia or cancer. Several other studies reported similar levels of sensitivity and specificity for differentiating between healthy, dysplastic, and malignant oral mucosa. Typical sensitivities and specificities ranged between 80–90% and 85–98%, respectively [71–73].

Other studies have utilized direct analysis of OCT scan profiles, rather than image-based criteria, as a means of delineating the site and margins of oral cancer lesions [70]. Using numerical parameters from A-scan profiles as diagnostic criteria, the decay constant in the exponential fitting of the OCT signal intensity along the tissue depth decreased as the A-scan point moved laterally across the margin of a lesion. Additionally, the standard deviation of the OCT signal intensity fluctuation increased significantly across the transition region between the normal and abnormal portions. The authors concluded that such parameters may well be useful for detecting and mapping the margins of oral cancer lesions. Such a capability has huge clinical significance because of the need to better define excisional margins during surgical removal of oral pre-malignant and malignant lesions.

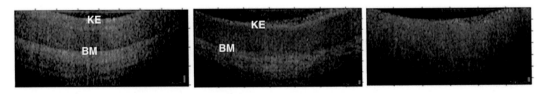

Fig. 7 OCT images of the oral mucosa. (**a**) healthy mucosa; (**b**) dysplastic mucosa; and (**c**) squamous cell carcinoma. BM-basement membrane; KE-keratinized epithelial surface. Note that (**c**) shows breakdown of basement membrane and surface keratinized layer of the epithelium. (Courtesy P.W.S.)

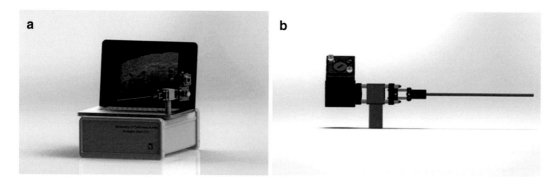

Fig. 8 Low-cost OCT system. (**a**) Imaging system. (**b**) Imaging probe. (Courtesy E.A. Heidari; reprinted with permission obtained by P.W.S.)

Several groups have applied innovative engineering techniques to reduce the cost of OCT technology and improve its affordability for dental clinicians and non-specialists. For example, a recent study in remote underserved villages in India utilized a prototype OCT system (Fig. 8) that was constructed at 10% of the cost of typical existing commercial systems [74–76]. The investigators also developed and tested an automated diagnostic algorithm which was directly linked to an image processing App. The automated cancer screening platform differentiated between healthy vs. dysplastic vs. malignant tissues with a sensitivity of 87% and a specificity of 83% vs. the histopathological gold standard [74–76].

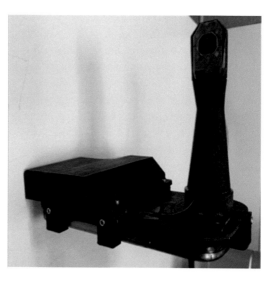

Fig. 9 Smartphone snap-on oral cancer probe. (Courtesy P.W.S.)

View to the Future

It is our opinion that the face of clinical instrumentation is changing rapidly. Smartphones and connectivity are becoming available worldwide, providing the opportunity to access remote and underserved patients and collect information with regard to high-risk behaviors, as well as signs and symptoms.

Smartphone-Based Autofluorescence Probe

White light images are readily available through inbuilt camera optics; fluorescence imaging is provided by means of a simple smartphone snap-on, plug-in, or Bluetooth-linked device. An ongoing study in India has demonstrated excellent oral cancer screening and management performance by such a device, linked to remote specialist access and equipped with a cloud-based triage algorithm. Inbuilt calendaring options allow for routinized monitoring and surveillance [77, 78]. Figure 9 shows the second-generation prototype which was one of the device configurations investigated in these studies and provided diagnostic sensitivities and specificities approximating 92–95% to distinguish between healthy vs. dysplastic and malignant oral mucosa [77, 78]. Currently, convolutional neural networks are being trained to add artificial intelligence-enabled discriminatory capabilities to the system, and the subject base is being expanded to include all types of oral lesions. In future, we envisage implementation of this type of approach by non-specialist field workers; perhaps patients might eventually even be able to upload photos that they themselves record for transfer to specialists as a means of facilitating oral cancer follow-up and management.

High-Resolution Fiberoptic Microendoscope

Several groups have mapped out to varying degrees the concept of a smartphone-based fiberoptic microendoscope for high-resolution fluorescence imaging [79–81]. Targeting autofluorescence or a signal enhanced by an exogenous fluorophore such as topical application of 0.01% proflavine, successful in vivo imaging and resolution of individual nuclei was reported. This capability would allow in vivo identification of the qualitative and quantitative differences between normal and precancerous or cancerous tissues. Such a portable, inexpensive device would be a useful tool to assist in the identification of early neoplastic changes in epithelial tissues at the point-of-care in low-resource settings.

Conclusion

The science and the benefits of novel imaging approaches for improving the detection and management of oral pre-cancer and cancer are very diverse. At this time, such imaging approaches all serve as adjuncts to the standard of care: expert clinical examination, risk factor assessment, and histopathology. However, as these various approaches continue to be tested and optimized, it is our hope that some aspects of oral cancer screening, diagnosis, monitoring, and management can be downstreamed to persons and technologies that are more readily accessible to the high-risk populations which typically have little access to specialist care.

References

1. Control of oral cancer in developing countries. A WHO meeting. Bull World Health Organ. 1984;62(6):817–30.

2. http://www.worldlifeexpectancy.com/cause-of-death/oral-cancer/by-country/.

3. Ries LA, Eisner MP, Kosary CL, et al., editors. SEER cancer statistics review, 1975–2002. Bethesda: National Cancer Institute; 2005. http://seer.cancer.gov/csr/1975_2002/citation.html.

4. Chaturvedi AK, Engels EA, Pfeiffer RM, et al. Human papillomavirus and rising oropharyngeal cancer incidence in the United States. J Clin Oncol. 2011;29:4294–301.

5. Amagasa T. Oral premalignant lesions. Int J Clin Oncol. 2011;16(1):1–4.

6. Mortazavi H, Baharvand M, Mehdipour M. Oral potentially malignant disorders: an overview of more than 20 entities. J Dent Res Dent Clin Dent Prospects. 2014;8(1):6–14.

7. Silverman S Jr, Gorsky M, Lozada F. Oral leukoplakia and malignant transformation. A follow-up study of 257 patients. Cancer. 1984;53(3):563–8.

8. Axell T, Pindborg JJ, Smith CJ, van der Waal I. Oral white lesions with special reference to precancerous and tobacco-related lesions: conclusions of an international symposium held in Uppsala, Sweden, May 18-21 1994. J Oral Pathol Med. 1996;25:49–54.

9. Kaugars GE, Burns JC, Gunsolley JC. Epithelial dysplasia of the oral cavity and lips. Cancer. 1988;62:2166–70.

10. Agarwal AK, Sethi A, Sareen D, Dhingra S. Treatment delay in oral and oropharyngeal cancer in our population: the role of socio-economic factors and health-seeking behaviour. Indian J Otolaryngol Head Neck Surg. 2011;63:145–50.

11. WHO. http://ocf.org.in/mainconfig.aspx?Moduleid=107&isexpandable=True&categoryid=162. Accessed 9/10/2017.

12. McGurk M, Chan C, Jones J, O'Regan E, Sherriff M. Delay in diagnosis and its effect on outcome in head and neck cancer. Br J Oral Maxillofac Surg. 2005;43(4):281–4.

13. Dolan RW, Vaughan CW, Fuleihan N. Symptoms in early head and neck cancer: an inadequate indicator. Otolaryngol Head Neck Surg. 1998;119(5):463–7.

14. Vernham GA, Crowther JA. Head and neck carcinoma: stage at presentation. Clin Otolaryngol Allied Sci. 1994;19(2):120–4.

15. Yao M, Epstein JB, Modi BJ, Pytynia KB, Mundt AJ, Feldman LE. Current surgical treatment of squamous cell carcinoma of the head and neck. Oral Oncol. 2007;43:213–23.

16. Neville BW, Day TA. Oral cancer and precancerous lesions. CA Cancer J Clin. 2002;52:195–215.

17. Ford PJ, Farah CS. Early detection and diagnosis of oral cancer: strategies for improvement. J Cancer Policy. 2013;1:e2–7.

18. Farmer P, Frenk J, Knaul FM, et al. Expansion of cancer care and control in countries of low and middle income: a call to action. Lancet. 2010;376:1186–93.

19. Petersen PE. The world Oral health report 2003: continuous improvement of oral health in the 21st century—the approach of the WHO Global Oral health

Programme. Community Dent Oral Epidemiol. 2003;31(1):3–23.

20. Amarasinghe HK, Usgodaarachchi US, Johnson NW, Lalloo R, Warnakulasuriya S. Public awareness of oral cancer, of oral potentially malignant disorders and of their risk factors in some rural populations in Sri Lanka. Community Dent Oral Epidemiol. 2010;38:540–8.

21. Paderni C, Compilato D, Carinci F, Nardi G, Rodolico V, Lo Muzio L. Direct visualization of oral-cavity tissue fluorescence as novel aid for early oral cancer diagnosis and potentially malignant disorders monitoring. Int J Immunopathol Pharmacol. 2011;24(2 Suppl):121–8.

22. Betz CS, Stepp H, Janda P, Arbogast S, Grevers G, Baumgartner R. A comparative study of normal inspection, autofluorescence and 5-ALA-induced PPIX fluorescence for oral cancer diagnosis. Int J Cancer. 2002;97:245–52.

23. Lingen MW, Kalmar JR, Karrison T, Speight PM. Critical evaluation of diagnostic aids for the detection of oral cancer. Oral Oncol. 2008;44:10–22.

24. Sharwani A, Jerjes W, Salih V, MacRobert AJ, El-Maaytah M, Khalil HS, Hopper CJ. Fluorescence spectroscopy combined with 5-aminolevulinic acid-induced protoporphyrin IX fluorescence in detecting oral premalignancy. J Photochem Photobiol B. 2006;83(1):27–33.

25. Lane PM, Gilhuly T, Whitehead P, Zeng H, Poh CF, Ng S, Williams PM, Zhang L, Rosin MP, MacAulay CE. Simple device for the direct visualization of oral-cavity tissue fluorescence. J Biomed Opt. 2006;11(2):024006.

26. Hanken H, Kraatz J, Smeets R, Heiland M, Assaf AT, Blessmann M. The detection of oral pre malignant lesions with an autofluorescence based imaging system (VELscope TM)—A single blinded clinical evaluation. Head Face Med. 2013;9:23.

27. Koch FP, Kaemmerer PW, Biestergeld S, Kunkel M, Wagner W. Effectiveness of autofluorescence to identify suspicious oral lesions—a prospective, blinded clinical trial. Clin Oral Investig. 2011;15:975–82.

28. Rana M, Zapf A, Kuehle M, Gellrich NS, Eckardt AM. Clinical evaluation of an autofluorescence diagnostic device for oral cancer detection: a prospective randomized diagnostic study. Eur J Cancer Prev. 2012;21:460–6.

29. Marzouki HZ, Tuong Vi Vu T, Ywakim R, Chauvin P, Hanley J, Kost KM. Use of fluorescent light in detecting malignant and premalignant lesions in the oral cavity: a prospective, single-blind study. J Otolaryngol Head Neck Surg. 2012;41(3):164–8.

30. McNamara KK, Martin BD, Evans EW, Kalmar JR. The role of direct visual fluorescent examination (VELscope) in routine screening for potentially malignant oral mucosal lesions. Oral Surg Oral Med Oral Pathol Oral Radiol. 2012;114(5):636–43.

31. Babiuch K, Chomyszyn-Gajewska M, Wyszyńska-Pawelec G. Use of VELscope for detection of oral potentially malignant disorders and cancers. Med Biol Sci. 2012;26:11–6.

32. Mehrotra R, Singh M, Thomas S, Nair P, Pandya S, Nigam NS, Shukla P. A cross-sectional study evaluating chemiluminescence and autofluorescence in the detection of clinically innocuous precancerous and cancerous oral lesions. J Am Dent Assoc. 2010;141(2):151–6.

33. Hanken H, Kraatz J, Smeets R, Heiland M, Assaf AT, Blessmann M, Eichhorn W, Clauditz TS, Gröbe A, Kolk A, Rana M. The detection of oral pre- malignant lesions with an autofluorescence based imaging system (VELscope™)—a single blinded clinical evaluation. Head Face Med. 2013;9:23.

34. Patton LL, Epstein JB, Kerr AR. Adjunctive techniques for oral cancer examination and lesion diagnosis: a systematic review of the literature. J Am Dent Assoc. 2008;139:896–905.

35. De Veld DC, Witjes MJ, Sterenborg HJ, Roodenburg JL. The status of in vivo autofluorescence spectroscopy and imaging for oral oncology. Oral Oncol. 2005;41:117–31.

36. Onizawa K, Saginoya H, Furuya Y, Yoshida H. Fluorescence photography as a diagnostic method for oral cancer. Cancer Lett. 1996;108:61–6.

37. Schantz SP, Kolli V, Savage HE, Yu G, Shah JP, Harris DE, Katz A, Alfano RR, Huvos AG. In vivo native cellular fluorescence and histological characteristics of head and neck cancer. Clin Cancer Res. 1998;4:1177–82.

38. http://media.denmat.com/OrchestraCMS/a2S800000001TjqEAE.pdf.

39. Yu B, Shah A, Nagarajan VK, Ferris DG. Diffuse reflectance spectroscopy of epithelial tissue with a smart fiber-optic probe. Biomed Opt Express. 2014;5(3):675–89.

40. Schwarz RA, Gao W, Redden Weber C, Kurachi C, Lee JJ, El-Naggar AK, Richards-Kortum R, Gillenwater AM. Noninvasive evaluation of oral lesions using depth-sensitive optical spectroscopy. Cancer. 2009;115(8):1669–79.

41. McGee S, Mirkovic J, Mardirossian V, Elackattu A, Yu CC, Kabani S, Gallagher G, Pistey R, Galindo L, Badizadegan K, Wang Z, Dasari R, Feld MS, Grillone G. Model-based spectroscopic analysis of the oral cavity: impact of anatomy. J Biomed Opt. 2008;13(6):064034.

42. Roblyer D, Kurachi C, Stepanek V, Williams MD, El-Naggar AK, Lee JJ, Gillenwater AM, Richards-Kortum R. Objective detection and delineation of oral neoplasia using autofluorescence imaging. Cancer Prev Res (Phila). 2009;2(5):423–31.

43. Wang A, Nammalavar V, Drezek R. Targeting spectral signatures of progressively dysplastic stratified epithelia using angularly variable fiber geometry in reflectance Monte Carlo simulations. J Biomed Opt. 2007;12(4):044012.

44. Arifler D, Schwarz RA, Chang SK, Richards-Kortum R. Reflectance spectroscopy for diagnosis of epithelial precancer: model-based analysis of fiber-optic probe designs to resolve spectral information from epithelium and stroma. Appl Opt. 2005;44(20):4291–305.

45. Georgakoudi I, Sheets EE, Müller MG, Backman V, Crum CP, Badizadegan K, Dasari RR, Feld MS. Trimodal spectroscopy for the detection and characterization of cervical precancers in vivo. Am J Obstet Gynecol. 2002;186(3):374–82.

46. Marina OC, Sanders CK, Mourant JR. Effects of acetic acid on light scattering from cells. J Biomed Opt. 2012;17(8):085002.

47. Dodeigne C, Thunus L, Lejeune R. Chemiluminescence as diagnostic tool. A review. Talanta. 2000;51:415–39.

48. Awan KH, Morgan PR, Warnakulasuriya S. Assessing the accuracy of autofluorescence, chemiluminescence and toluidine blue as diagnostic tools for oral potentially malignant disorders—a clinicopathological evaluation. Clin Oral Investig. 2015;19(9):2267–72.

49. Epstein JB, Silverman SJ, Epstein JD, Lonky SA, Bride MA. Analysis of oral lesion biopsies identified and evaluated by visual examination, chemiluminescence and toluidine blue. Oral Oncol. 2008;44:538–44.

50. Ram S, Siar CH. Chemiluminescence as a diagnostic aid in the detection of oral cancer and potentially malignant epithelial lesions. Int J Oral Maxillofac Surg. 2005;34:521–7.

51. Awan KH, Morgan PR, Warnakulasuriya S. Utility of chemiluminescence (ViziLite™) in the detection of oral potentially malignant disorders and benign keratoses. J Oral Pathol Med. 2011;40:541–4.

52. Oh ES, Laskin DM. Efficacy of the ViziLite system in the identification of oral lesions. J Oral Maxillofac Surg. 2007;65:424–6.

53. McIntosh L, McCullough MJ, Farah CS. The assessment of diffused light illumination and acetic acid rinse (Microlux/DL) in the visualisation of oral mucosal lesions. Oral Oncol. 2009;45:e227–31.

54. Sharma N, Mubeen. Non-invasive diagnostic tools in early detection of oral epithelial dysplasia. J Clin Exp Dent. 2011;3:E184–8.

55. Huber MA, Bsoul SA, Terezhalmy GT. Acetic acid wash and chemiluminescent illumination as an adjunct to conventional oral soft tissue examination for the detection of dysplasia: a pilot study. Quintessence Int. 2004;35:378–84.

56. Epstein JB, Gorsky M, Lonky S, Silverman S Jr, Epstein JD, Bride M. The efficacy of oral lumenoscopy (ViziLite) in visualizing oral mucosal lesions. Spec Care Dentist. 2006;26:171–4.

57. Farah CS, McCullough MJ. A pilot case control study on the efficacy of acetic acid wash and chemiluminescent illumination (ViziLite) in the visualisation of oral mucosal white lesions. Oral Oncol. 2007;43:820–4.

58. Kerr AR, Sirois DA, Epstein JB. Clinical evaluation of chemiluminescent lighting: an adjunct for oral mucosal examinations. J Clin Dent. 2006;17:59–63.

59. Kennedy JC, Pottier RH. Endogenous protoporphyrin IX, a clinically useful photosensitizer for photodynamic therapy. J Photochem Photobiol B. 1992;14(4):275–92.

60. Cassas A, Fukuda H, Battle A. Hexyl ALA ALA-based photodynamic therapy in epithelial tumors: in vivo and invitro models. Proc SPIE. 2002;3909:114–23.

61. Leunig A, Rick K, Stepp H. Fluorescence imaging and spectroscopy of 5-aminolevulinic acid induced protoporphyrin IX for the detection of neoplastic lesions in the oral cavity. Am J Surg. 1996;172(6):674–7.

62. Ebihara A, Liaw L-H, Krasieva TB. Detection and diagnosis of oral cancer by light-induced fluorescence. Lasers Surg Med. 2003;32(1):17–24.

63. Leunig A, Mehlmann M, Betz C. Detection of squamous cell carcinoma of the oral cavity by imaging 5-aminolevulinic acid-induced protoporphyrin IX fluorescence. Laryngoscope. 2000;110(1):78–83.

64. Leunig A, Mehlmann M, Betz C. Fluorescence staining of oral cancer using a topical application of 5-aminolevulinic acid: fluorescence microscopic studies. J Photochem Photobiol B. 2001;60(1):44–9.

65. Chang CJ, Wilder-Smith P. Topical application of photofrin for photodynamic diagnosis of oral neoplasms. Plast Reconstr Surg. 2005;115(7):1877–86.

66. Nitin N, Rosbach KJ, El-Naggar A, Williams M, Gillenwater A, Richards-Kortum RR. Optical molecular imaging of epidermal growth factor receptor expression to improve detection of oral neoplasia. Neoplasia. 2009;11:542–51.

67. Huang D, Swanson EA, Lin CP. Optical coherence tomography. Science. 1991;254:1178–81.

68. Tsai MT, Lee HC, Lee CK, Yu CH, Chen HM, Chiang CP, Chang CC, Wang YM, Yang CC. Effective indicators for diagnosis of oral cancer using optical coherence tomography. Opt Express. 2008;16(20):15847–62.

69. Wilder-Smith P, Lee K, Guo S, Zhang J, Osann K. In-vivo diagnosis of oral dysplasia and malignancy using optical coherence tomography: preliminary studies in 50 patients. Lasers Surg Med. 2009;41:353–7.

70. Tsai MT, Lee CK, Lee HC, Chen HM, Chiang CP, Wang YM, Yang CC. Differentiating oral lesions in different carcinogenesis stages with optical coherence tomography. J Biomed Opt. 2009;14(4):044028.

71. Hamdoon Z, Jerjes W, Al-Delayme R, McKenzie G, Jay A, Hopper C. Structural validation of oral mucosal tissue using optical coherence tomography. Head Neck Oncol. 2012;4:29.

72. Lee CK, Chi TT, Wu CT, Tsai MT, Chiang CP, Yang CC. Diagnosis of oral precancer with optical coherence tomography. Biomed Opt Express. 2012;3:1632–46.

73. Jerjes W, Upile T, Conn B, Betz CS, Abbas S, Jay A, et al. Oral leukoplakia and erythroplakia subjected to optical coherence tomography: preliminary results. Br J Oral Maxillofac Surg. 2008;46:e7.

74. Heidari E, Sunny SP, James BL, Lam T, Tran AV, Ravindra DR, Uma K, Praveen BN, Wilder-Smith P, Chen Z, Suresh A, Kuriakose MA. Utilizing optical coherence tomography to assess oral cancer malignancy in a low resource setting. SPIE Photonics West, San Francisco, CA, January 28–February 2, 2017.

75. Tran AV, Lam T, Heidari E, Sunny SP, James BL, Kuriakose MA, Chen Z, Birur PN, Wilder-Smith P. Evaluating imaging markers for oral cancer using optical coherence tomography. Lasers Surg Med. 2016;48(4). Late breaking abstracts #LB29.

76. Sunny SP, Heidari AE, James BL, Ravindra DR, Subhashini AR, Keerthi G, Shubha G, Uma K, Kumar S, Mani S, Kekatpure V, Praveen BN, Suresh A, Lam T, Wilder-Smith P, Chen Z, Kuriakose MA. Field screening for oral cancer using optical coherence tomography. American Head and Neck Society (AHNS) 9th International Conference on Head and Neck Cancer, Seattle, WA, July 16–20, 2016.

77. Firmalino V, Anbarani A, Islip D, Song B, Uthoff R, Takesh T, Liang R, Wilder-Smith P. First clinical results: optical smartphone-based oral cancer screening. 38th American Society for Laser Surgery and Medicine Annual Meeting, Dallas, TX, April 11–15, 2018.

78. Takesh T, Anbarani AG, Ho J, Firmalino V, Liang R, Wilder-Smith P. A novel low-cost miniature probe for oral diagnosis. Lasers Surg Med. 2017;49(4). Late Breaking Abstracts #LB26.

79. Shin D, Pierce MC, Gillenwater AM, Williams MD, Richards-Kortum RR. A fiber-optic fluorescence microscope using a consumer-grade digital camera for in vivo cellular imaging. PloS One. 2010;5:e11218. https://doi.org/10.1371/journal.pone.0011218.

80. Rahman MS, Ingole N, Roblyer D, et al. Evaluation of a low-cost, portable imaging system for early detection of oral cancer. Head Neck Oncol. 2010;2:10. https://doi.org/10.1186/1758-3284-2-10.

81. Skandarajah A, Sunny SP, Gurpur P, Reber CD, D'Ambrosio MV, Raghavan N, et al. Mobile microscopy as a screening tool for oral cancer in India: a pilot study. PLoS One. 2017;12(11):e0188440. https://doi.org/10.1371/journal.pone.0188440.

Index